Public Trust in Medical Research?

Ethics, law and accountability

Philip Cheung BA(Bio.Sc.), MA(Ed), PhD

Visiting Research Fellow
Marie Curie Hospice, Newcastle
Honorary Fellow
Department of Anthropology, University of Durham

W0234902

 **CRC Press**
Taylor & Francis Group
Boca Raton London New York

CRC Press is an imprint of the
Taylor & Francis Group, an **informa** business

First published 2007 by Radcliffe Publishing

Published 2016 by CRC Press
Taylor & Francis Group
6000 Broken Sound Parkway NW, Suite 300
Boca Raton, FL 33487-2742

ISBN-13: 978-1-84619-179-4 (pbk)

Visit the Taylor & Francis Web site at
http://www.taylorandfrancis.com

and the CRC Press Web site at
http://www.crcpress.com

British Library Cataloguing in Publication Data

A catalogue record for this book is available from the British Library.

Typeset by Phoenix Photosetting, Chatham, Kent

Contents

Preface

As a lay person with a knowledge of science and philosophy and experience in education in the NHS and in higher education, culminating with academic research experience, I can comment on the subject of medical research from various standpoints. In addition as a result of working as a member of the NHS Retained Organs Commission I have had the opportunity of coming into contact with a large number of members of the public and many members of the medical profession. Some of the discussion in this work is therefore grounded in personal experiences provided by the public. Such materials could provide a stimulus for lay people and professionals to engage in further deliberations. If this is achieved, then my aim of encouraging the public to be proactive in determining the future agenda for medical and medical research could be realised.

It is highly probable that people will forget history and major events which do not touch them personally even though at the time they can sympathise. The documentary evidence in this book regarding a historical practice of the medical profession which went ethically astray will serve to remind the public it would be unwise to help perpetuate the idea that professionals know best. The personal accounts and the findings from various official inquiries offer learning materials for students in various academic disciplines. It is hoped that students and practitioners will learn from past history and that their professional attitudes will be shaped by people's painful experiences.

Laws and codes of conduct are necessary for just a few in society but collectively we are responsible for what happens in society. It is difficult when a community within a profession is under attack because of bad practice. It will seem unjust for those good practitioners to be similarly judged. Inevitably the image of the good practitioners is tarnished in the process. The cases highlighted in this book demonstrate the importance of taking collective ethical responsibility in the practice of one's profession.

Evidence of how laws governing medical practice and medical research in the previous centuries were framed provides an insight into how legislators might have been influenced by professional pressure and consequently laws were made against the public interest.

Shaping the future for medicine and medical research is everyone's responsibility. The education sector, legal system, academic and research communities and the professions involved should take corporate responsibility for ensuring that ethical laws are incorporated into professional practice. The public can exert more influence than in the past by being more inquisitive about biomedical inventions. The key to success is that the public and the medical profession should establish a healthy partnership.

Philip Cheung
May 2007

About the author

Philip Cheung currently holds the post of Visiting Research Fellow at Marie Curie Hospice, Newcastle Upon Tyne, responsible for research and development in palliative care research. He is an Honorary Fellow of the Department of Anthropology of the University of Durham. He is a Trustee of the Newcastle Citizens Advice Bureau.

He has recently set up a lay research group in Newcastle encouraging informal carers to become involved in palliative care research. His role in this group is to help lay people understand research issues and to facilitate them to initiate their own research in palliative care and use their research evidence to influence practice.

He is an experienced advocate. As a member of the NHS Retained Organs Commission during April 2001–March 2004, he was particularly involved in working with distressed families. As a researcher he also sought to introduce public opinion surveys that aimed to enhance the Commission's understanding of the issues surrounding organ retention following post-mortem examinations.

While at Durham University during 1994–2004, he specialised in health-related research. In particular he worked with many secondary and primary schools on smoking prevention which attracted a great deal of media interest. He was awarded a Royal Society grant to implement a peer-tutoring project in 2001 involving secondary school and primary school pupils.

Dedication

This book is dedicated to those parents and families in the UK who have been affected by some of the events described in this book.

I pay particular tribute to the grieving parents and families, especially those who have had to bury their children and relatives more than once.

I value the experience of working with members of PITY II and other support groups.

Perhaps this book will encourage those who have been involved in campaigning for change and who have given up so much of their time to help and support others.

Chapter 1

Medical progress and human costs

Issues of medical progress

If we look back over the last four decades, medicine has given hope to many people and saved many lives primarily as a result of a better understanding of diseases, due partly to a rapid advancement in biochemistry and biotechnology and the ability of the physicians and surgeons to develop new treatments and innovative surgical techniques. The advancement in biochemistry and biotechnology in particular has contributed to a range of innovative medical treatments including the possibility of conquering some of the genetically inherited conditions. It has been claimed by fertility experts that embryos can be screened for 6000 diseases, thereby the risk of x-linked diseases can be minimised by 'cherry picking' male embryos that do not carry the abnormal gene. If medical scientists continue to strive for cures, genetic aberrance in humans could be a phenomenon of the past.

Medical science has made advances into childlessness. For example, the *in vitro* fertilisation technique or IVF has conquered the problem of infertility. Eggs can now be frozen for women who desire to delay their motherhood. Researchers in Newcastle upon Tyne, UK, have been able to grow sperm from mouse embryonic stem cells and use them to fertilise eggs, resulting in seven mice being born. In due course, the new technique developed by the Newcastle team may be applied to treat male infertility problems. The possibilities are limitless.

One can safely say that most, if not all, innovative medical and surgical treatments are underpinned by painstaking research, including the development of new drugs, which has played a significant role in the management and control of the disease process. During the course of these scientific developments, members of the public are directly or indirectly involved either as donors to, or as recipients of, a new surgical procedure. For example, prior to the introduction of heart valve replacement surgery as a safe practice in the early 1960s, heart valves were salvaged from the deceased for technical and experimental purposes. Once the technique was perfected, many patients benefited from freeze-dried homografts obtained from healthy hearts of deceased persons. Since then, the transplantation of major organs has been mastered and with the help of immunosuppressive drugs, organ transplantation of heart, lungs and liver can now be offered as a safe surgical procedure. Scientists have now turned their attention to using embryonic stem cells (ESCs) obtained from a person for the manufacture of whole organ autograft, which could be a real alternative as donor organs are in short supply.

While we can celebrate the success of medical science, should we not also critically examine some of these developments against specific criteria or principles and in the light of public opinion? One of the questions that needs addressing is whether there are human costs associated with medical advancements. Consider for example, the first-in-man clinical trials[1] carried out by Parexel, a contract research organisation, in March 2006. (The term 'first-in-man trials', 'first-in-man studies', 'first-in-man clinical trials' and 'Phase One clinical trials' of high-risk medicines are used by the Expert Scientific Group on Phase One Clinical Trials, interchangeably.) Eight healthy volunteers were used for the trial. Six of them were given the untested drug TGN1412, which is a monoclonal antibody developed for the treatment of chronic inflammatory or immune conditions such as rheumatoid arthritis and leukaemia.[1] Within minutes of the drug administration, a violent allergic reaction, referred to scientifically as a cytokine release, occurred and the six healthy volunteers were left fighting for their lives.

The technique of culturing or cloning antibodies was developed in the late 1970s. It involves injecting a mouse or other type of animal with a particular allergen, i.e. the mouse is immunised and a range of antibody-producing cells is triggered as a result. These antibody-producing cells normally die after a few divisions, so are not useful for producing large quantities of antibodies. But if a specific antibody-producing cell from the immunised animal is combined with a myeloma cell – an immune system cancer – then the fused cell when cultured in a special medium can produce large quantities of antibodies.[2]

It might seem reasonable for a doctor to offer a treatment of unproven efficacy to a sick person with a limited life span in exchange for a possible recovery or a better quality of life. On the other hand, is it reasonable to subject healthy people to unknown risks as in the TGN1412 trial? If the six healthy volunteers had died as a result of the trial, the costs to the families would be incalculable, even though the experiment was carried out in the name of medical science. Is there a compromise between medical progress and human costs? One might suggest that if individuals are unwilling to make sacrifices, progress in medical research could be seriously jeopardised and more people will suffer in the long term.

Limits of medicine and medical research

Some of us seem not to be content with the notion that the human body has a natural lifespan and are reluctant to face the reality of death and the pursuit of immortality becomes a human obsession. Advancements in science and medicine tend to give the impression that immortality can be within our grasp. It was thought 30 years ago that someone suffering from coronary thrombosis would have to be content with the prognosis, i.e. the person would succumb to the disease. Now, coronary bypass surgery is a well-developed technique and the survival rates after bypass surgery are high. The technique of replacing a diseased heart has been perfected and many patients continue to live for an extended period. Surgeons are now able to perform multiple organ transplantations providing donor organs are available. The public may gain the impression that spare-part surgery is an essential service provided by the health service alongside other more mundane services such as geriatric care and community care for the mentally ill. The doctors who are specialising in this field of surgery will want to achieve the impossible by, for example, multi-system surgery, with the help of pharmaceutical products conquering the biochemistry of tissue rejection.

Human society, at least in the developed world, is reluctant to accept the inevitability of dying. Dying could be considered as part of the human growing process. Is it good medicine and ethical to use considerable amounts of money to extend lives, sometimes putting the patient through an assault course in the process, in return for postponing death? Should some of the health service resources be reallocated to those who are old and infirm, to those who are mentally ill, to try to improve their quality of life? Chronic geriatric and psychiatric medicine in particular are seen as less prestigious fields of practice. Since the health service is strapped for cash, and transplantation surgery is often carried out at the expense of other branches of medical practice such as orthopaedics, geriatric or community medicine, should resource distribution in the health service be re-examined? Should the principle of resource allocation be based on fairer distribution, that is, should funds be allocated to medical interventions and treatments where the greatest numbers will benefit in society? Is there an ethical dimension to the use of National Health Service (NHS) resources?

The Department of Health pledged to double kidney transplants and increase heart and lung transplants by 10% by 2006. However, the targets are unlikely to be met as the current trend shows that at the end of March 2006, 6698 people were still waiting for transplants, a 9% increase compared to the previous year. There was a decrease of 9% in heart and heart/lung transplants compared to the previous year.[3] Those who are in the field of transplantation surgery expressed their anxiety, particularly following the Alder Hey, Bristol and other organ scandals. The Department of Health has an obligation to encourage more donors to come forward otherwise this life-saving technique is at serious risk. It seems to me that one needs to take stock of the current technology-based medicine and consider its real value against other significant health needs.

To give life to another person through organ donation is a praiseworthy act. Donor organs normally come from largely healthy persons whose life is suddenly cut short, usually due to a road traffic accident, head injury or suicide for example. They may also come from someone who is in a vegetative state, which is described as 'someone living like a vegetable, without will or consciousness; functioning involuntarily',[4] i.e. in a state of human non-being. This human non-being state can be maintained for as long as necessary by mechanical means until suitable recipients are found for transplantation. When suitable recipients are found the life of the human person artificially kept alive can be ended at will by a team of competent surgeons. Is this ethically permissible? Is this a decent death? A couple of views from those who have experienced organs being given for transplantation show how complicated are the issues in practice.

> A 64-year-old man speaking of his wife, stated: 'She had never died. She died when the organs were donated.'

> A mother in her late forties consented to her daughter's organs being used for transplantation. She later explained: 'To me, donating meant killing my child.'
>
> (Notes from author's personal diary)

The message given by the above individuals touches the affective aspect rather than mechanical aspect of organ donation. The scientists and doctors are looking at the human body from the usefulness point of view. It is an object worthy of being salvaged. From the donor relatives' point of view, they are talking about a person with a unique presence prior to becoming brain-dead. The human suffering associated with the advancement in transplant surgery can be inestimable for the deceased's relatives. There is no human compensation from their point of view even through altruism. Though this may not be the only or indeed the 'normal or standard' reaction, since there are relatives who have spoken positively of the psychological aspect of donation, it is important evidence of the emotional, human and ethical situation for some individuals.

Consideration of the method used by clinicians in obtaining donor organs for transplantation surgery from the relatives of a person in a vegetative state and the emotional aspects of giving described above are not intended to deter individuals from such an act, rather to raise awareness of the serious human effect that may follow. Perhaps many of us have not even given such a matter any serious attention. Sometimes emotions overcome reason when such a decision is put to us. How does one react to such a request when it occurs?

There is in general avoidance of talking about death and dying, a subject that it is not comfortable to discuss at home, in schools or in hospitals. Opportunities are rarely provided even in a religious setting. Even those whose training or background qualify them as experts see death and dying as taboo. Death is the fate of humanity and yet it is not well understood. If one were to adopt Galen's notion that the human body is a machine and able to be repaired, then the idea of immortality would be a real possibility, at least in terms of bioscience and medicine. Human immortality then becomes a scientific challenge. Should medicine be primarily concerned with prolonging life even if the limits are stretched? What about those who are in need of terminal care? Assisting someone to die peacefully and with dignity should be seen as being as praiseworthy as saving a life. Why are doctors and scientists so obsessed with conquering death?

Major events in recent years such as the Bristol Royal Infirmary Inquiry into children's post-operative death following cardiac surgery, the Royal Liverpool Children's Hospital Inquiry into organ retention (Alder Hey) following postmortems and the Inquiry into the removal and retention of adult brains for research brought about by Cyril Isaacs' widow (these events will be discussed in Chapter 5) provided a platform for a long-awaited public debate regarding the essence of specific medical practices and the basic philosophy of medicine and medical research. They have provided an opportunity for interested members of the public and society in general to examine some of the basic human values inherent in medical practice and research which we, as users of the health service, care deeply about.

The Alder Hey, Bristol and Isaacs families have been asking many of the same basic questions as faced by philosophers and other thinkers. For example, the families have provoked us to explore more deeply the issues of human society and human practices, particularly in the world of medicine. They challenge the idea of human existence, our place in the world, the meaning of life and, like the theologians and philosophers, they ask questions about death as well as life. The biologists and medical scientists have also been challenged as they confront the belief which seems sometimes to be held by some researchers that the body is merely made up of a bag of genes. More fundamentally, they are delving into the very root of basic human values governing human practices in society: the existence and purpose of rules in human society and what rules exist and to what extent these rules should help curb individual selfishness and inclinations. The whole notion of scientific progress in the name of common good has been seriously challenged.

Daniel Callahan, Director of International Programmes at the Hastings Center in Garrison, New York, a centre that has five research programmes specialising in ethics and scientific research, spoke a few years ago to the Nobel Laureate, Joshua Lederberg, on the issue of medical research. In his article 'When science is just another good cause', published in the *New Scientist*, he recalled the remark made by Lederberg: 'Those who do not support medical research will have the blood of those who die on their hands.'[5] Lederberg's claim might sound melodramatic but similar claims have also been made by some doctors and pathologists involved in organ retention as justification for continuing a widespread inappropriate and unlawful medical practice that has brought a great deal of unnecessary human suffering.

Whenever families in Liverpool and elsewhere in the UK asked why doctors and pathologists needed to take everything from the child's body, the reply was that the organs retained would help the study of genetic diseases or other rare conditions. The implication is that without these organs doctors would not be able to help others and that anyone who raised objections to organ retention would be subjected to Lederberg's emotional blackmail. Lay people might find the rehearsed argument from doctors difficult to resist. Even those with doubts, or who had reached a different point of view after much thought, might feel they ought to be persuaded.

A statement was made at the Chief Medical Officer's Summit in January 2001 by a former CMO about the importance of having access to archive collections of organs. He said: 'HIV and AIDS, variant CJD, certainly could not have been recognised without access to such collections.'[6] This might have an element of reality but how many people have actually benefited? How much have all those collections contributed when measured against the outrage of the families concerned? How will the findings help those who have contracted these incurable diseases? In general, not just in relation to organ and tissue matters, does medicine pursue agendas that end up with a credit balance in medical gains versus any damage to individuals along the way or from side effects? A more pertinent question might be whether medical research should give more attention than it does to the origin of iatrogenic conditions, as there is evidence to correlate oral polio vaccine with the development of HIV/AIDS[7] and the natural form of pituitary growth hormone with variant CJD.[8] The pharmaceutical industry is understandably prepared to defend its methods of development of drugs and vaccines on the grounds that 'it had a moral obligation to do the expensive research that would cure disease and relieve suffering.'[5]

Is medical science going astray?

Recently, the public has been made aware of the important development of cloning technology in the study of neurological conditions such as Alzheimer's and Parkinson's and other inherited conditions. Previously, samples of affected cells had to be taken from living patients which could put them at risk. By using cloning technology, the diseased cells can be created outside the patient's body and therefore the behaviour of the diseased cells can be studied without having to wait for the patients to develop their symptoms. Thus the scientists can be a step ahead of the disease process and many people could be saved from such debilitating conditions. Cloning can also be used to develop and test new drugs without having to use animals and human subjects.

This new scientific innovation sounds convincing, but what happens when innovation goes astray? Is there any guarantee that cloning will be used only to good purpose and with safety? Callahan suggests researchers engaged in novel research, such as in embryonic stem cells, would defend their position by saying that 'there was an ethical duty to pursue a line of study that could eventually save thousands, even millions, of lives',[5] but sees such an argument as 'a misuse of what can be called the research imperative...which can be understood as a striking manifestation of the human desire to know and to use science to improve the human condition. But like a number of good things that can go sour if we do not take care, it is a claim that can act as a kind of moral and social bully.'[5] If we think of moral sensibility, in part, as a manifestation in a particular era of 'normal' everyday concerns, then the use by this writer of the word 'bully' is interesting since in so many walks of life bullying is a cause of disquiet.

The most radical potential use of human cloning technology is to treat inherited diseases, particularly those affecting whole organs such as the lungs which can be replaced by methods using stem cells. It would also solve many of the problems that have recently plagued gene therapy such as the risk of causing cancer.[9] Clearly, human cloning research requires strict ethical and legal supervision. The consequences could be on the same scale as seen when the remarkable advances of Einstein's great generation of scientists led to the dropping of the atomic bomb. It seems a huge and fanciful leap from human cloning issues to Einstein and atomic bombs, but the argument demonstrates an assumption of omniscience by those involved in scientific research.

Let us consider the steps by which a new potential human being may be created by this means for the study and treatment of disease. Firstly, *in vitro* fertilisation is a technique for creating an embryo whereby an egg is fertilised by a sperm outside the human body. I am in agreement with those who think that the embryo so created should be considered as a 'potential person' (*see* reference 10 for use of this expression in a different context) with the capacity for developing to full term. Note that during the initial stage of *in vitro* application, more than one embryo is created so as to have a greater chance of a successful result, thus creating several 'potential persons'. The cells from the newly created embryo(s), commonly known as embryonic stem cells (ESCs), will be subject to genetic engineering whereby the diseased gene(s) will be removed and replaced by selected disease-free genes so that at the end of the procedure every cell within the embryo is normal. Remaining cells and embryos will be stored or subsequently destroyed, if permission is given by the donors concerned, when the scientists decide that the embryos have no further use. A nucleus from one of the ESCs is introduced into an egg taken from a woman. The final step is to implant the 'healthy' embryo with the correct gene into a woman's womb and allow it to develop into a baby.

The child developed by the process described above is a cloned child, but is also a new individual with new genes derived from the egg and the sperm of a woman and a man. This new child with a new set of genes is produced through therapeutic cloning, which is different from reproductive cloning described below. Therapeutic cloning avoids the feature of natural selection that allows certain recessive genes which carry disease to be passed on from generation to generation.

A cloned child from one of its parents can be produced using the same technique as described previously, using material from one of its parents. This is known as reproductive cloning. Here too, reproductive cloning differs from the process of natural selection, in that the genes for the reproductively cloned child are artificially selected for specific purposes. Reproductive cloning could be regarded as a form of human eugenics where the most profitable genes will be selected from one human individual. The end result of reproductive cloning if it were conducted on a large scale would be to achieve a 'perfect' human population where individuals within the population would have the same genes, e.g. for blue eyes, fair hair or other preferred genes.

Reproductive cloning brings with it a number of social and moral issues. If the development were allowed to be conducted totally unchecked, an artificially developed gene pool could be established within the human population. Reproductive cloning can be construed as interference with nature and as restricting the development of human diversity which is generally viewed by humanity as a human characteristic to be appreciated and sustained. Historically, in some communities with a restricted migratory pattern, inherited diseases, such as diabetes, and mental disabilities, were more common. One can imagine the long-term health and social consequences of selective 'inbreeding' engineered by reproductive cloning if the strictest control is not exercised.

At present, the Human Fertilisation and Embryology Authority supports the concept of therapeutic cloning with the proviso that it is carried out ethically. Reproductive cloning is not legal in this country at present. However, in the future, the need for reproductive cloning might be so persuasive that politicians might be canvassed to engineer a policy whereby it is permitted in special circumstances. If the campaigners for reproductive cloning were to succeed, then the unique diversity of the human race could be replaced by a group of individuals with the same attitudes and behaviour.

Human cloning involves genetic engineering. Genes are manipulated in the laboratory. The chance of being successful relies heavily on the competence of the scientist as a technician since precise manual manipulation is required during the *in vitro* fertilisation. Damage can be caused to the cells during laboratory manipulation. If damage is caused to the cells then an abnormal potential being will be created. In which case, who would bear the moral responsibility for the malformed person if the embryo were allowed to develop to birth and beyond? How acceptable is it that the malformed potential human being (embryo), that has deliberately been created, be destroyed? Perhaps that is a different order of concern to that of destroying an embryo that is diseased or defective but naturally created. Each time some great potential advance in medicine or science comes into view some of us may say 'this goes too far'. We appear to stand opposed to progress. But does this mean we should not speak out? Will everything always be all for the best in the end? Will the sufferings of the first patients always, as in the case of transplants, be followed by success?

The cloned animal Dolly the sheep suffered from premature arthritis and lung disease and died prematurely in 2004. The Dolly the sheep project was partly funded by a pharmaceutical company interested in developing a new blood product for the treatment of lung diseases such as cystic fibrosis. An artificially created person could suffer the same fate as Dolly. Morally, who would be responsible for any unpredictable disease suffered by an 'actual person'[10] created either by therapeutic or reproductive cloning? In addition, to what extent would the person created by either means have the same chance as other individuals to enjoy life, bearing in mind the main purpose of the cloned person is to be used to save another life? What if the cloned person eventually objects to the prime purpose of his/her creation? Or if the cloned person's life span is cut short like Dolly's, would the scientist concerned be responsible for the death of his/her creation?

So far, the issue of informed consent has not been raised. In the case of human cloning, who could speak on behalf of a 'potential person' not yet designed? Will the parents speak on behalf of this unknown person, or the scientist in the laboratory?

During the latter part of 2005 there was the case of an American couple whose child suffered from a genetic blood disorder. The only way in which the diseased child's life could be saved was by means of therapeutic cloning. Once the cloned baby developed, then blood from the umbilical cord could be taken as soon as the cloned child was born. Samples of the cord blood would then be injected into the diseased child. If the treatment failed, would the cloned child be considered useless therapeutically? Would the child be subsequently labelled a failure? What would he/she be eventually told of the reasons for his/her actual existence?

Following successful treatment of their sick child the American couple had to face the difficult question of what ought to be done with the remaining embryos artificially produced during *in vitro* fertilisation, as described previously. The choice was stark. The remaining embryos could be allowed either to live or to be destroyed. If an embryo is considered to be a potential human being, then is it right to destroy a new life? What right does one have to destroy a potential human being? Parents who are driven to select therapeutic cloning as a means of saving another life are inevitably faced with this impossible dilemma. How could parents whose task in the first place was to sustain another life then choose to destroy lives? Some bioethicists do not necessarily accept that an embryo is a potential person with rights. It does not then however follow that if the embryo is not human or not yet human that the ethical problems are solved.

It is difficult to arrive at a consensus on the issues of human nature, even among philosophers, psychologists, theologians, biologists and social scientists. Some might even deny the existence of human nature. Professor Roger Trigg, in his book *Ideas of Human Nature: an historical introduction*, argues that human nature must exist as a real moral basis since thinkers such as Plato, Aquinas, Hobbes, Hume, Darwin, Marx and Freud argued about the same issues regarding humanity over a period of almost two and a half millennia.[11] The questions such thinkers ask about human nature may have even more relevance in the 21st century when society is faced by the ethical issues raised by modern biomedicine.

The International Red Cross defines humanity as 'protecting life and health and to ensure respect for the human being, promoting mutual understanding, friendship, co-operation and lasting peace amongst all peoples'.[12] The Red Cross is presumably led by practical people who may or may not be philosophers or ethicists. They presumably accept the notion of humanity quite easily and do not need deep thought about the need for respect for each other. They confront the problems created by war or natural disasters.

The *Catechism of the Catholic Church* has this to say about basic and applied research. It states that 'Basic scientific research, as well as applied research, is a significant expression of man's dominion over creation. Science and technology are precious resources when placed at the service of man and promote his integral development for the benefit of all. By themselves however they cannot disclose the meaning of existence and of human progress. Science and technology are ordered to man, from whom they take their origin and development; hence they find in the person and in his moral values both evidence of their purpose and awareness of their limits.'[13] The suggestion that science should recognise its own limits is one that is widely appreciated, not least by scientists themselves. The consequences of not wanting to contemplate its own limits could have unknown and undesirable consequences. The scientist who led the team that created Dolly, Dr Ian Wilmut, has been quoted as saying: 'Human cloning is finally here. I believe…cloning promises such benefits that it would be immoral not to do it. That is why a number of UK labs, including my own, plan to apply to the relevant authorities for permission to study human cloning here in the UK. And while I remain implacably opposed to cloning *per se*, I do envisage that producing cloned babies would be desirable under certain circumstances, such as preventing genetic diseases.'[9] But does such scientific endeavour have consequences for society? What benefits are there for mankind? What are the moral imperatives associated with such an undertaking?

The role of the public in shaping progress

On occasion one needs to speak out or raise objections against scientific developments if they are thought to be harmful to society. Human cloning is an example where such a social debate is needed. It would be difficult to rectify what might go wrong. Therefore, if we have serious concerns, should we not raise objections to its application? Again, the choice is stark: we can either remain silent or speak out against it. Is neutrality a real choice? The *Catechism of the Catholic Church* asserts that 'it is an illusion to claim moral neutrality in scientific research and its applications… Science and technology by their very nature require unconditional respect for fundamental moral criteria. They must be at the service of the human person…'[13] Of course this assertion is orientated towards Catholic teachings or at least to the view of nature widely shared by Europeans for centuries. It provides a basis for open and transparent discussions about medical science and interventions.

There is a tendency to look up to medicine and medical research as we are naturally influenced by more positive aspects. Unfortunately, the less positive side is often hidden and in some cases forgotten. For example, how many of the younger generation remember the devastating consequences of thalidomide and the associated suffering that was caused to many families? Thalidomide was prescribed by doctors in the 1960s for pregnant women as an anti-sickness agent, resulting in some women giving birth to grossly deformed children. (The term 'deformity' is described in the Medical, Nursing and Allied Health

Dictionary as 'a condition of being distorted, disfigured, flawed, malformed or misshapened, which may affect the body in general or any part of it. It may be the result of disease, injury or birth defect.')[14] In this context we are referring to some people who were born with only limb stubs or other forms of severe birth defects.

The consequences of thalidomide are carried by those individuals who were born with gross deformities and by those who care for them. You are only reminded of the consequences which were brought about by pharmaceutical discovery and medical prescribing when a victim is seen. Similarly, antibiotics were regarded as wonder drugs following their discovery during the Second World War. However, due to over-prescribing, methicillin-resistant *Staphylococcus aureus* (MRSA) is now one of the more common causes of death after surgery or following hospital admission. When these iatrogenic problems surface they are often overshadowed by other more interesting, glamorous and emotive new discoveries such as new cancer drugs or treatments, the success of *in vitro* fertilisation and the miracle of organ transplant.

There is a danger that people may over-react when things go wrong in science and medicine and when a particularly distasteful event takes place. There is no denying that human suffering would be far greater without the knowledge and skills of doctors and other health professionals. However, the frontiers of medicine seem to have moved beyond natural human limits. Scientists appear sometimes to determine their own agenda without giving serious attention to possible moral or social objections. Currently, society seems unable to control the development of science or to exercise due scrutiny over what scientists do in their laboratories.

Medicine and medical research should in principle assist in the 'promotion of the integral good of the human person, in keeping with the unique dignity which is ours by virtue of our humanity. Consequently, it is evident that every medical procedure performed on the human person is subject to limits; not just the limits of what is technically possible, but also limits determined by respect for human nature itself, understood in its fullness: what is technically possible is not for that reason alone morally permissible.'[15] The public need to remember this maxim when faced with the views of the scientific community.

References

1 Department of Health. Expert Scientific Group on Phase One Clinical Trials – Interim Report. London: Department of Health; 2006.
2 Voet D, Voet J. *Biochemistry*. 2nd ed. New York: John Wiley & Sons, Inc; 1995.
3 UK Transplant. Transplant save lives. [accessed October 2006]. Available from: http://www.uktransplant.org.uk/ukt/statistics.jsp.
4 MacNalty AS. *British Medical Dictionary*. London: Caxton Publishing Company; 1961.
5 Callahan D. When science is just another good cause. *New Sci*. 2004; **181(2436):** 18–19.
6 Department of Health. Chief Medical Officer's Summit: proceedings. Computer-aided transcription by Harry Counsell and Co. London: Department of Health; 2001; 33.
7 Hooper E. *The River: a journey back to the source of HIV and AIDS*. London: Allen Lane, The Penguin Press; 1999.
8 BBC. CJD fears over growth hormone [accessed 2002]. Available from: http://news.bbc.co.uk/1/hi/health_notes/98757/stm.

9 Wilmut I. The moral imperative for human cloning. *New Sci.* 2004; **181(2435):** 16–17.

10 Glover J. *Causing Death and Saving Lives*. Harmondsworth: Penguin Books; 1987.

11 Trigg R. *Ideas of Human Nature: an historical introduction*. Oxford: Basil Blackwell; 1988.

12 International Red Cross. Proclamation of the fundamental principle of the Red Cross [accessed August 2006]. Available from: www.icrc.org/web/eng/siteeng0.nsf/htmlall/ 5mje9n.

13 Catechism of the Catholic Church. London: Chapman; 1999: 486–95. Reproduced by kind permission of Continuum of International Publishing Group.

14 Mosby S, Anderson KN, editors. *Medical, Nursing and Allied Health Dictionary*. St. Louis Missouri: Mosby-Year Book Inc; 1998: 453.

15 Pope John Paul II. Special address by His Holiness John Paul II. Transplantation Proceedings. 2000; **33:** 31–2.

Chapter 2

What is good and ethical medicine?

The practice of medicine is fundamentally good (the word 'good' is used in an ordinary language sense here), but does this mean that everything the doctor does is also ethical? The same question also applies to medical research. If we consider a situation where a teenage person seeks medical assistance from her general practitioner (GP) for an abortion, the choice for the GP is a difficult one. It would seem unkind and unethical to the teenage girl if the doctor refuses to help because of his/her own moral standards. However, if the doctor decides to help, then the decision would be deemed by some as unethical as medical assistance is being given to terminate a potential life. Yet, from the point of view of the teenage girl, it is a good decision as her personal dilemma and social difficulties are solved. So the action taken by the GP could be regarded as good and ethical from the patient's point of view.

What is good medicine? Does good practice equate with ethical practice? The previous chapter queries whether what is acceptable in medical practice is necessarily ethical and the consequences for medical science if it is allowed to go unchecked. The public, on the whole, is not arguing against the importance of medical and scientific research, rather it is questioning the means by which the ends are achieved. Those who question should not be dismissed as naïve or ill-informed. They are not Luddites. It is of course sometimes difficult for lay people to assess the reasonableness of any medical and scientific research as there is often insufficient information available for such a judgement to be made. The conclusions drawn by lay people often rely on emotion and the apparent benefit disclosed by the research communities. For example, one would agree that *in vitro* fertilisation (IVF) has satisfactorily solved the clinical problems for many previously childless women or couples. However, it can also bring false expectation and major disappointment for some. More importantly, the application of IVF also raises a number of long-term social policy and ethical issues. For example, is it the inalienable right of every woman to have a child? Is surrogacy an appropriate way of bringing a new human being into the world, and what are the social and personal consequences for that individual? Are there reasonable objections to fertilised eggs being commercialised? Lay contributions may not produce answers, but they help ensure that necessary questions are not overlooked.

Many discoveries in medicine in the past have made significant contributions to the understanding and treatment of diseases, but are the means by which the results were attained necessarily ethical? For example, Pasteur in 1878 argued the case for the germ theory of infection. He postulated that micro-organisms were responsible for disease, putrefaction and fermentation, that only particular organisms could produce specific conditions, and once organisms were known prevention would be possible by developing vaccines. While Pasteur was investigating the cure for cholera and anthrax, he experimented with animals such as chickens, goats and cattle. His idea of prevention is long lasting as we are still benefiting from his work. The animal rights campaigners would consider Pasteur's work in retrospect unethical. Here is the obvious essential difficulty. Nothing is gained by judging the past from the present. But lessons can be learned.

We have benefited from the results of Pasteur's scientific work in the treatment of rabies. However, Pasteur could be severely criticised since he administered untested vaccine to two boys who were dying from the disease. Fortunately the boys were saved. Later, Pasteur injected the untested vaccine into another 2000 people worldwide as a preventive measure. The efficacy of the vaccine had not been proven, even though it was successfully tested on chickens, goats and cattle. Criticism could be levelled at Pasteur as he was injecting healthy people with an unproven vaccine. Whether full consent was sought from the healthy volunteers is not known (probably it was not). Was that an ethical undertaking?

There are many other notable examples which demonstrate the fine line between good and ethical pursuit of knowledge and cures and unacceptable practice. Edward Jenner injected an apparently healthy boy with untested cowpox vaccine in order to find a cure for smallpox. His vaccine has largely eradicated the disease throughout the world.

The Australian pathologist Howard (later Lord) Florey (1898–1968) shared the Nobel Prize with Ernest Chain and Alexander Fleming for the discovery of penicillin. Florey launched a project on micro-organism antagonism. From mould, he developed a drug similar to penicillin which was tested successfully on mice. Later, he tried it on a dying policeman who had succumbed to an infection after pricking himself while pruning roses. Although it helped to combat the infection initially, the policemen later died since insufficient amounts of pure therapeutic substance could be extracted from the mould.

In the examples of Pasteur, Jenner and Florey it is relatively easy to determine whether they were justified in pursuing their cause as the ends appear to justify the means, that is, lives have been saved and the benefit has been shown to be universal. In which case, should one be too concerned about the way in which the results were attained? Does it really matter how many animals were killed in the process? Does it matter if a small number of humans were subjected to potential risks or even death? Should one be interrogating the social and ethical consequences of humans being used as guinea pigs so long as the outcome helps sustain life? These questions can be further examined by using another example: the discovery of the polio vaccine.

No one would argue that the successful introduction of oral polio vaccine in the 1960s has achieved almost worldwide eradication of a fatal condition. Therefore, its introduction can be regarded as good science and good medicine. However, if one were to examine the experimental process against the principles of the Nuremberg Code and other research rules, discussed in the next chapter, would one regard the development of the polio vaccine as ethical? A particular team of doctors and scientists in the 1950s decided to feed oral polio vaccine to humans for the first time. There were gaps in the knowledge concerning the mechanism of infection and immunity in poliomyelitis due to the fact that human beings had never been exposed to actual administration of living poliomyelitis virus for clinical trial purposes.[1] The trials involved using non-immune human volunteers for the first time in February 1950. The living poliomyelitis virus was previously administered to animals but yielded conflicting results.[1] Volunteer number one was a six-year-old boy so severely handicapped that he had to be fed the vaccine through a stomach tube, which suggests that he himself was most unlikely to have volunteered for this or any other experiment. The other nineteen volunteers were similarly handicapped, but there is no mention anywhere about permission being either sought or granted from the respective parents.[2]

It has also been reported that during the process of vaccine development, mentally defective patients in the Congo were deliberately infected with faeces contaminated with the poliomyelitis virus and then brought together with those living in the same hospital who had not been infected.[1] Was this ethical practice? The terms 'mentally handicapped' and 'mentally defective' were used by the author of *The River* to mean persons who lack the mental capacity to make informed decisions regarding medical experimentation such as the oral vaccine experiment conducted in 1950. The term 'mentally handicapped' was used until the 1980s for people with less than what was considered normal IQ when it was changed to 'people with learning disability'. The latter term encompasses many conditions such as dyslexia, autism, etc. In the context of the oral polio vaccine experiment, the children used were mentally handicapped which highlights the questionable ethical conduct of the researchers.

Good medical practice and biomedical research conduct require doctors and scientists to think ethically. Today's researchers, thinking ethically, would not be able to overlook the ethical concerns associated with the use of mentally defective children, as previously described, irrespective of country of origin. They might not ignore the more demanding ethical issues in the polio experiment, and they might not accept that the end always justifies the means or that the good of the greatest number in society justifies harm to individuals. It would be the failure to think ethically in our time that would allow practices that contravene basic human values.

There can be no disagreement about the huge advances brought about by Pasteur, Jenner and other scientists that have benefited human society so greatly. The questions about ethics may suggest that 'pure' morality based on universal absolute values may not be realistic, and that there should be a different ethical regime in different circumstances and in different eras. However, thinking about those great achievements, and then about recent events such as the illegal medical practice of removing and retaining organs at post-mortem examination, suggests that universal ethics are needed as a guide at all times in research. Perhaps what is needed is to encourage students in medicine, in law and in other healthcare professions to think about universal ethics through education and training, and the careful framing of laws and professional codes so that there is the best possible convergence of ethics and utilitarianism.

What is good and what is ethical? Some philosophers would suggest that something good is essentially ethical. Plato said goodness is the name of a 'form' which exists separately from the perceptual world since goodness itself does not depend on the nature of our world and certainly is not dependent for its validity on human judgements, and is unaffected by human belief.[3] Take, for instance, honesty as a form of goodness in all circumstances; it is not subject to change and it exists independently of human judgement and belief. In this sense, goodness is an ideal at which one should aim.

To be an ethical person is the same as being a good person. Kant wrote that in making an ethical decision you should believe that the principle of your thinking is suitable to constitute not just what is right in the case, but in all cases. The emphasis of Kant in this sense is man's freedom to act in accordance with universal laws of nature and of morals.[4] If one were to apply Plato's and Kant's philosophies in medical practice and research, the doctor must think for himself but at the same time think from the standpoint of everyone, but also think consistently. These rules prevent human individuals from making errors based on biases, personal desire and idiosyncrasies.

The problem may be that the real meaning of 'good' has been lost due to common usage. The word 'good' is often used colloquially, i.e. have a good time, have a good party, etc. A research project using stolen brains could be classified within the scientific circle as a good piece of scientific enquiry as it might help to identify the causes of Alzheimer's, thereby new solutions might be found to treat people suffering from this degenerative condition. Surely theft is neither good nor right, even if the intended aim was to do good. Right and wrong form the balance weighed up in ethics. If good and ethical can be used interchangeably, then what is good must be ethical.

To return to the example of oral polio vaccine, one might judge from the scientific standpoint that the polio vaccine experiments were scientifically a good approach as appropriate laboratory procedures had been followed and the results have been applied positively throughout the world. Ethically, was it right or wrong to deliberately exploit mentally handicapped people in the Congo when there were significant risks attached to the use of living poliomyelitis virus?

The principal researcher of the oral polio vaccine programme was unwilling to disclose openly in his seminar paper the status of his first 20 volunteers, leading to a suspicion that there was no intention to seek consent from them. They were merely described as volunteers. The only clue to their identity was that some, including the very first volunteer, had had to be fed through stomach tubes. In fact, the participants were described as 'feeble-minded children',[1] judged to be incompetent in making informed decisions even if they were permitted to do so. Today we would say that the children were coerced into taking part. Was that ethical? Was it enlightened practice?

The lesson to be learned is that doctors and researchers should be encouraged to think ethically. To denounce or punish those who in the past seem to have acted unethically is less useful than the recognition of the need to think ethically today. Do scientists and doctors in fact think differently now from the way they thought in the past? The problem is that ethics is constant, but the thinking and application of ethical principles by doctors and scientists is reactive to clinical and scientific issues. The latest suggestion on stem cell research is that palliative care patients can be subjects for clinical trials prior to studies carried out on animals which is described by the research community as the *in vitro* development in animals model. Therefore, can one be optimistic about biomedical science having a constant ethical framework which is followed by all?

There are many other examples in medicine that raise questions about research ethics. For example, from 1959 the use of growth hormone extracted from the pituitary gland was a good and novel approach for stunted children. The correlation between growth hormone treatment and the development of

Creutzfeldt-Jakob disease (CJD) among those treated became known in the 1980s. The treatment was ended in the UK in 1985 following the death of a US patient. It has now come to light that '34 out of 1900 people who had received the natural form of the hormone had died of CJD in the UK'.[5] The number of patients treated by the natural form of human growth hormone who might eventually contract CJD cannot be known until new cases are diagnosed.

It has also been estimated that the risk of CJD associated with blood transfusion could reach up to 60 000 UK recipients a year.[6] Medicine and science do not have perfect vision into the future. Maybe the problem can be classed as one of quality control. Where was the proper analysis of potential hazards? Maybe from the start there was ethical uncertainty about a treatment developed to improve the quality of life, which was so novel that all the attendant factors could not be easily assessed.

No one would want to disparage the development of new drugs as it has a global significance for the prevention, control and management of diseases. But in some cases, the application of life-saving drugs raises some uneasy ethical dilemmas. The current postcode lottery system operating in the UK, where only some hospital trusts can afford certain treatments, would be regarded as unethical as there is the issue of inequality within the same system of healthcare. AIDS affects the unborn, children and adults in Africa and in other poorer countries of the world. The disease has resulted in millions of people dying prematurely and leaving many children orphaned, with long-term inestimable social and economic consequences for these countries. In the West drugs are available to AIDS sufferers and yet the populations in the developing world are denied these life-saving remedies. 'Good' medicine cannot be said to be necessarily ethical.

References

1   Hooper E. *The River: a journey back to the source of HIV and AIDS*. London: Allen Lane, The Penguin Press; 1999; 204–17.

2   Koprowski H, Jarvis GA, Norton TW. Immune responses in human volunteers upon oral administration of a rodent-adapted strain of poliomyelitis virus. *Am J Hyg*. 1952; **55**: 108–26.

3   Plato. *The Republic*. Lee D. (trans.) London: Penguin Books; 1955.

4   Kant I. *Groundwork of the Metaphysics of Morals*. Paton HJ, tr. New York: Harper Torchbooks; 1948.

5   BBC. CJD fears over growth hormone [accessed 2002]. Available from: http://news.bbc.co.uk/1/hi/health/s002489.stm.

6   Alternative Health Directory. CJD and blood transfusion [accessed 2002]. Available from: http://alternativehealth.co.uk/nexart2/page2.html.

Chapter 3

The role of ethics in medical research

Ethics and the health professionals

Every action that one takes has a positive and negative aspect which might or might not have consequences for others. For example, if one takes a holiday just to please oneself then there are no conflicting interests so long as one is happy in taking time off. However, if a gardener in a drought-declared location chooses to water his garden then there are consequences for his immediate neighbour as well as for the rest of the region in which he resides. This example might be benign as it does not really have any major consequences for the people around him except that he is being inconsiderate, antisocial and selfish. Is selfishness a bad attribute? Are there criteria that govern what is good or bad?

During one's working life there are many occasions where one has to weigh up the pros and cons of each situation that confronts us. For example, an AIDS research worker in Africa is confided in by one of his colleagues who has been diagnosed as being HIV positive. The worker is faced with the dilemma of whether the information passed on to him should be made known to the colleague's family. Once the information has been disclosed his colleague might be faced with the strong possibility of being isolated from his family and his community. If the information given to him by his colleague remains undisclosed then there might be undesirable health consequences for the community as the disease could be spread unnoticed. Perhaps the prime factor governing the decision here is how many people could be affected in the future if the information is kept away from the community. A suitable alternative needs to be chosen. It is a good attribute to value a friendship, but when this interferes with the notion of common good, as shown by the situation above then one is left with no suitable alternative but to choose to protect the health of the community. Can one be judged to be unethical?

Ethics provide a set of rules which govern standards of human behaviour. Ethical rules enable us to determine in a general sense what is right, what is wrong, and what is acceptable or unacceptable. These rules should be regarded as generally immutable otherwise erroneous judgements will be made on occasions. For example, honesty is seen by Plato as a form of goodness valid in all circumstances; it is not subject to change and it exists independently of human judgement and belief.[1] In fact, among philosophers from even before Plato's time to the present there has been a debate between those who think that in practice values such as honesty are defined in a way that is context based and those who think they are defined in a way that is absolute. If values are context based, there could be many variations in the way we interpret honesty or other human basic values such as kindness, compassion, decency, etc.

Withholding information when asked by patients or relatives, or telling lies for fear of causing further distress to the patient's relatives, may be seen by doctors as being protective towards the public. This generally adopted attitude is referred to by the medical profession as medical paternalism and doctors by and large do not believe that there is anything wrong with the practices associated with such an attitude. (Medical paternalism will be further discussed in Chapter 11). If honesty or truth is accepted as an ethical value then avoiding the truth for fear of upsetting the patient or telling lies is simply unethical. Philosophers such as Plato would simply point out that lying is the opposite of truth. If ethics is seen in this sense, subjective application of these rules is not permissible.

People from every walk of life are governed by these rules. Ethical rules do not have a social class boundary or pertain to the interests of groups within society. By implication these rules also govern our working life and individuals are held responsible for their own actions. The practice of medicine is governed by the Hippocratic Oath, which should be seen as setting out the moral imperatives for medical practitioners. If these imperatives are not adhered to in professional practice, serious professional wrongdoing will result.

We have witnessed a miscarriage of justice where Sally Clark was wrongfully convicted in November 1999 of smothering 11-week-old Christopher in December 1996 and shaking eight-week-old Harry to death in 1998. She was jailed for life. Two members of the medical profession, the medical expert witness, Professor Sir Roy Meadow and the Home Office prosecution pathologist, Dr Alan Williams, were implicated. Roy Meadow was recognised as an expert renowned for his work in cot deaths. He made fundamental errors when he presented his statistical calculations in Clark's case where he claimed the occurrence of two cot deaths in one family is extremely rare: 'the odds are 1 in 73 million.' He gave evidence in a string of other court cases including those of Angela Cannings and Trupti Patel. In 2002, the president of the Royal Statistical Society challenged Roy Meadow's calculations.[2] In January 2003 'Professor Meadow's evidence was discredited by three appeal judges.'[3] In addition, Dr Alan Williams, the prosecution Home Office pathologist, was found to have withheld vital evidence from the court. In the light of these findings, Mrs Clark was subsequently released from jail in June 2003. Both doctors were found guilty of serious professional misconduct and were struck off from the medical register by the General Medical Council.

It is difficult to explain the behaviour of these two doctors. Why did Roy Meadow give fallacious evidence in court? Why did the Home Office pathologist withhold information from the court when he was under oath? One plausible explanation might be Roy Meadow wanted to prove his theory even though it was believed to be wrong by other scientists. Alternatively, both doctors had the intention to deceive. According to Plato and Kant, both actions are bad.[1,4]

There are some extreme cases where a doctor has completely disregarded ethics and laws. The paediatric pathologist at Alder Hey (the Royal Liverpool Children's Hospital), Professor van Velzen, was implicated in the Alder Hey organ scandal. The serial killer, Harold Shipman, a general medical practitioner, was arrested on 7 September 1998 and charged with the murder of Mrs Grundy and with other offences associated with the forgery of her will. In January 2000, Dr Shipman was convicted of the murder of 15 of his patients and of forging the will of one of them. An independent inquiry was established by the government in January 2001, chaired by Dame Janet Smith. The first report confirmed that Shipman had killed 215 of his patients over a period of 24 years.[5]

Ethics provide an absolute moral framework for all actions irrespective of circumstances. If we agree that ethics provide universal permanency for all things and in all circumstances then there is no possibility of anyone interpreting ethical rules flexibly. If one holds the belief that it is wrong to terminate a life as it is against the ethical and moral code then it is wrong to kill a fellow human being, irrespective of the circumstance in which one finds oneself and even if a doctor believes terminating a patient's life would ease unnecessary suffering.

There is a tendency for some to think that the rules of ethics could be rewritten. Instead of thinking about how the rules of ethics might be changed, it would be more constructive to contemplate how the rules of ethics ought to be strictly applied in specific situations. A recent example will support this argument. In November 2006, the Royal College of Obstetricians and Gynaecologists convinced the Nuffield Council on Bioethics working group to consider the ethics of euthanasia for the sickest of newborn babies. The inquiry is now looking into 'the ethics of prolonging life in fetuses and the newborn'.[6] The newborns in this case are those who are the sickest or the most profoundly disabled. The college ethics committee 'tells the inquiry it feels euthanasia has to be considered and debated for completion and consistency sake...if life-shortening and deliberate interventions to kill infants were available, they might have an impact on obstetric decision-making, even preventing some late abortions...'[6] Is this a reasonable request from those who practise medicine? The request from the College of Obstetricians and Gynaecologists should be viewed as a desire to change the ethical basis of medical practice against the background of unchecked medical advancements as described in Chapter 1. Surely, the debate should be focused on the need to provide palliative care for these unfortunate newborn babies and to provide support for their parents.

Bodies such as the Nuffield Council on Bioethics, the General Medical Council and government departments could be influenced and persuaded from time to time to rewrite practice rules which impinge on ethics. There is a real danger that the new rules governing medical practice could be driven by changing social circumstances, rather than being ethically based.

Government departments and professional bodies concerned with professional regulation seem unable to reflect the constancy of ethical rules. It seems that the regulatory framework can be redesigned from time to time following crises or professional scandals such as the ones referred to earlier in this chapter. For example, the system of medical regulation was last reviewed in the early 1970s following 'a crisis of confidence in the General Medical Council on the part of the medical profession. Through the 1970s, 1980s and early 1990s, the system of medical regulation again faced mounting criticism, much of it focusing on the failure to identify early, and deal effectively with, doctors who were a danger to their patients.'[7] As a result of the disclosure at Liverpool and elsewhere of the wrongful removal and retention of human organs by doctors, the General Medical Council instigated reforms, resulting in the construction of a new government framework for regulation of medicine that put the safety of patients first.[8] The new General Medical Council declaration states that good medical practice is the 'explicit statement of duties, responsibilities, values and standards for doctors, based on a strong public and professional consensus about the qualities that are important'.[9]

The examples of the Home Office pathologist involved in giving evidence in Sally Clark's prosecution case, van Velzen's organ scandal in Liverpool and Harold Shipman in Manchester not only highlight the fact that ethical rules cannot guarantee the good conduct of individual medical practitioners but also show that there are ethical issues in collective governance within a profession. Professional bodies responsible for regulating practice have an ethical and legal duty to protect the public and if patients are harmed due to the ineffectiveness of the regulatory machinery then, in principle, the professional bodies concerned should bear some responsibility for any wrongdoing.

The report *Good Doctors, Safer Patients*, commissioned by the Secretary of State for Health, following the publication of the fifth report of the Shipman Inquiry, reiterated Dame Janet Smith's serious criticism of the General Medical Council. It said that Dame Janet Smith was 'highly critical of the General Medical Council, concluding that its culture, membership, methods of working and governance structures were too likely to support the interests of the doctors rather than to protect patients'.[7] Should the ethical issues raised by Dame Janet Smith be further debated by the medical profession and by society as a whole?

The report cited above proposes a major programme of reform including monitoring doctors' performance. How much confidence can one have in the new system? Dame Janet condemned weaknesses and dysfunctions in past systems for protecting patients from harm and cast serious doubt on the effectiveness of the proposals for the five-yearly revalidation of a doctor's licence to practise. In particular, she criticised the proposed reliance on the annual appraisal of NHS doctors, judging it not to constitute a true evaluation of the full range of a doctor's performance and delivery of care and thus an ineffective method of detecting doctors who are incompetent, dysfunctional or delivering care to a poor standard.[7]

The Hippocratic Oath may be seen by some as needing updating, but the essence of the oath should remain the same for all times and for all circumstances. Patient-centred care should always be one of the moral imperatives for doctors and other health professionals. One might suggest that instead of revising the framework for evaluating doctors' performance, one should seriously examine the way in which the essence of the Hippocratic Oath is put into practice, and how doctors might be closely monitored against the criteria set out therein.

Ethical imperatives governing medical research

The conduct of medical and biomedical research is also governed by rules. For example, the 10 key directives in the Nuremberg Code[10] should be seen as the rules for the conduct of human experimentation. It is important to point out that the Nuremberg Code was formulated after the atrocities that took place in the Nazi concentration camps came to light after the Second World War. The Code was created to prevent researchers from abusing human subjects.

The Code states that:

1 The voluntary consent of the human subject is absolutely essential. This means that the person involved should have legal capacity to give consent; should be in a situation as to be able to exercise free power of choice, without the intervention of any element of force, fraud, deceit, duress, over-reaching or other ulterior form of constraint or coercion and should have sufficient knowledge and comprehension of the elements of the subject matter involved as to enable him to make an understanding and enlightened decision. …The duty and responsibility for ascertaining the quality of the consent rests upon each individual who initiates, directs or engages in the experiment. It is a personal duty and responsibility which may not be delegated to another with impunity

2 The experiment should be such as to yield fruitful results for the good of society, unprocurable by other methods or means of study, and not random and unnecessary in nature

3 The experiment should be so designed and based on the results of animal experimentation and knowledge of the natural history of the disease or other problems under study that the anticipated results will justify the performance of the experiment

4 The experiment should be so conducted as to avoid all unnecessary physical and mental suffering and injury

5 No experiment should be conducted where there is an *a priori* reason to believe that death or disabling injury will occur, except perhaps in those experiments where the experimental physicians also serve as subjects

6 The degree of risk to be taken should never exceed that determined by the humanitarian importance of the problem to be solved by the experiment

7 Proper preparation should be made and adequate facilities provided to protect the experimental subject against even remote possibilities of injury, disability or death

8 The experiment should be conducted only by scientifically qualified persons

9 During the course of the experiment the human subject should be at liberty to bring the experiment to an end if he has reached the physical and mental state where continuation of the experiment seems to him to be impossible

10 During the course of the experiment the scientist in charge must be prepared to terminate the experiment at any stage.

The Nuremberg Code provides a set of ethical imperatives for medical researchers. However, the Code cannot guarantee absolute ethical conduct as there are opportunities for varied interpretation or misinterpretation. Putting the Code into practice in its absolute sense requires the medical researchers to fully comprehend the statements contained in the Code and conscientious application of its principles when translated into practice.

If we examine the statements contained in the Nuremberg Code in turn, from the simple to the more complicated, Items 3, 4, 7 and 8 appear to be clear-cut and can be implemented without controversy. No medical researchers should want to jeopardise any scientific principles upheld by them as scientists, e.g. that any experiments so conducted must be based on sound knowledge and understanding of their own discipline. Neither should they want to subject any human beings to physical or mental suffering and injury. Item 8 can be easily implemented as it demands that medical experiments with human subjects can only be carried out by scientifically qualified persons.

With reference to Item 2 of the Nuremberg Code, how does one judge whether any experiment may be 'fruitful' for the good of society, and 'fruitful' in what sense? Are there specific criteria upon which researchers can make an ethical judgement when engaging in a human study, including clinical trials of medicinal products? Currently, medical scientists possess the knowledge and technology to screen embryos for specific genetic traits or defects. It is not unimaginable that in the future certain genetic characteristics such as criminality could be identified and screened, as in principle it would be good to have a crime-free society. In which case, a social policy could be driven by science and implemented under the guise of utilitarianism, requiring any embryo carrying that genetic tendency to be terminated during pregnancy. Would it be 'fruitful' for the good of society? Those who believe life begins after conception would regard such a policy as fundamentally wrong. The opponents of pro-life would perhaps praise the value of such a policy. Others who believe in the theory of nurturing might propose that instead of taking such a drastic social policy action, the characters of individuals who were born with such tendencies could be reshaped through education and appropriate family upbringing. Their pent-up energy could be channelled to good use. Which would be considered as a more appropriate way for scientists to determine whether an experiment is fruitful or not? Does interfering with the process of natural selection in human society comply with the Code?

Item 5 of the Nuremberg Code is an interesting one and ethically difficult to apply because if it is implemented in full it might deter scientists from experimenting with their fellow human subjects. Many scientific experiments will be stopped in their tracks if we believe there is an *a priori* reason that they could incur even a remote possibility of injury or death. Is there absolute certainty that human subjects being experimented upon with new medicines or surgical techniques will be protected against possible harm?

Item 9, at first glance, seems unambiguous as the human subjects participating in the experimental process can decide when to terminate the programme. However, there might be circumstances where the participants might not be in full control of their physical and mental well-being as shown in the TGN1412 untested drug trial (referred to in Chapter 1). How could these participants in the TGN1412 trial be able to terminate the trial when serious life-threatening complications have occurred or when the participants have lost consciousness?

The first rule in the Nuremberg Code is the most difficult to achieve. It emphasises the absolute necessity to obtain voluntary consent from those who are asked to commit themselves to scientific experiments which the individuals concerned have no knowledge of and where there are potential risks attached. The term 'absolute necessity' covers specifically the legal capacity of the individual to give consent; the individual rights to exercise free choice; the decision made at the end of the consent process must be based on sound understanding and free from deceit, fraud, duress, coercion. This rule stipulates that the duty of obtaining freely given consent cannot be delegated to another person by the researcher.

We have seen that some of these principles have been violated in the past as discovered by members of the public in Liverpool and elsewhere around the country where organs from the deceased were removed and retained without the knowledge of, and consent from, the relatives.

Fundamentally, the Nuremberg Code, if it is implemented fully and conscientiously, can protect vulnerable human subjects who are exposed to scientific experiments which are claimed to have potential benefits for society. Unfortunately, the Nuremberg Code has been superseded by the World Medical Association Declaration of Helsinki.[11] Item (ix) of the Declaration regarding consent states that: 'In any research on human beings, each potential subject must be adequately informed of the aims, methods, anticipated benefits and potential hazards of the study and the discomfort it may entail. He/she should be informed that he/she is at liberty to abstain from participation in the study and that he/she is free to withdraw his/her consent to participation at any time. The physician should then obtain the subject's freely-given informed consent, probably in writing.'

If Item (ix) of the Helsinki Declaration is compared with the first Nuremberg principle, there are immediate differences. There exist many loopholes in the Helsinki Declaration. The term 'adequately informed' can be disputed as it can be interpreted in different ways by different researchers, depending on their ethical behaviour. The Helsinki Declaration has removed some of the absolute values, such as free choice, self-determination, openness, honesty, and avoidance of using deceitful means, which were endorsed by the Nuremberg Code. It has also removed the imperative of 'ought' and replaced it by 'probable'. Surely, consent can only be valid if it is given in writing.

There are no intelligent explanations as to why the Nuremberg Code was replaced by the Helsinki Declaration. One possible explanation might be that those who were responsible for producing the Declaration might want to forget the atrocities which happened in the Second World War where human beings including children were subjected to harmful medical experiments. Alternatively, the Nuremberg Code might have been seen to be unfit for scientific purposes in the latter part of the 20th century and the 21st century. We should remember however that since its adoption in 1965 the Declaration has been amended in 1975, 1983 and 1989. The question that should be asked is why was it necessary to change the Declaration so frequently unless the revised rule was again seen as unfit for its purpose? Historically, when rules or laws, e.g. the abortion law, were seen to sit uncomfortably with the social climate of the time, professionals or politicians would be moved to initiate change. The fundamental question is can ethical rules that have stood the test of time be satisfactorily rewritten by a few individuals? How can Kant's maxim of 'all human actions must be based on reason and that any actions taken by a human person must be unconditionally good' be satisfactorily reformulated?

The replacement of the Nuremberg Code demonstrates the problem of updating rules and interpreting rules flexibly during the updating process. The rule governing consent becomes less watertight and liable to be used as an instrument for unethical application. The ambiguities that have been introduced into the Helsinki Declaration demonstrate very clearly the problems of reinterpreting ethical rules based on changed circumstances, bearing in mind that it has been amended several times.

Despite the universal condemnation of horrific experiments which took place during the Second World War, unethical medical research using human subjects continues. A report in *The Lancet* in 1997 revealed that the US Center for Disease Control had supported unethical trials of new drugs for the treatment of HIV in which a placebo group (a control group who were denied the new drugs or any other appropriate medications) of HIV-positive women were allowed to infect their children perinatally. Did these trials contravene the Nuremberg Code for human experimentation? What force do such codes have?

In addition to the Nuremberg Code and the Declaration of Helsinki,[11] medical and scientific research is also governed by other codes of conduct such as the Ethical Principles and Guidelines for the Protection of Human Subjects of Research,[12] the United Nations Convention on the Rights of the Child,[13] and the Human Rights Act 1998.[14]

The Helsinki Declaration emphasises not only the importance of informed consent, but the rights of those who are deemed legally incompetent (where physical and mental incapacity makes it impossible for them to give informed consent or where the subject is a minor).[11] Article 2 of the Human Rights Act 1998 stresses the 'right to life'; Article 5 refers to the 'liberty and security of the person'; Article 9 refers to the 'right of freedom of thought, conscience and religion'; Article 13 advocates the 'right to an effective remedy' and Article 14 supports the notion of the 'right to non-discrimination'.[14]

The Ethical Principles and Guidelines for the Protection of Human Subjects of Research relate specifically to 'respect for persons', 'beneficence', and 'justice'.[12] Respect for persons is governed by two ethical convictions, namely: (i) that individuals should be treated as autonomous agents, and (ii) that persons with diminished autonomy are entitled to protection. Autonomy refers to self-determination whereby a person should be able to exercise his/her personal liberty. When autonomy is applied to contemporary healthcare practice and research it focuses specifically on informed consent. Beneficence implies a duty to do good to others and that patients have a right to expect those with a duty of care towards them to be trustworthy. The Hippocratic maxim of 'do no harm' applies here and refers to both the proactive care as well as the measures which protect from additional harm. (The additional harm refers to Illich's theory of iatrogensis.[15]). It is the duty of the doctor to ensure that procedures, policies and protocols are designed to minimise the risks of physical and emotional injury. The last rule, 'justice', is to ensure that healthcare resources are used equitably.

There are a number of principles associated with the proper research use of human tissue. For example, the following considerations were proposed by the Health Council of the Netherlands. Is the intended use of human organs morally acceptable insofar as its purpose is to promote human health? Is the human tissue used with the greatest of care? Is the relationship between doctor and patient undermined by the use of body material? Can the patient rest safe in the knowledge that his/her own needs will continue to come first? Should people be forced to get involved in scientific experiments even if it is in a good cause? Has privacy been afforded to those whose material is put to further use? Is the material treated with respect and dignity? Has the principle of non-commercialisation been observed?[16]

Recently, in 2003, the Department of Health issued an interim statement concerning the use of human organs and tissues: 'The human body and its parts should be treated with respect and, in general, organs and tissue should be removed, retained or used only for purposes for which patients have had the opportunity to give their valid consent.'[17]

It must be emphasised that codes of practice governing research are not abstract frames of reference; they provide the absolute criteria necessary to distinguish between good and evil, right and wrong in the way experimentation is conducted and experimental subjects are treated in laboratory and clinical settings.

Ethics is not about exploring abstract ideas. It is a way of thinking seriously about our most important actions. Respect, for example, has a constant and permanent human value and should be given unconditionally when dealing with each other. Similarly, treating the human body, dead or alive, with reverence is an integral part of the human nature. If the idea of integrity is applied in a professional setting, it means that the person will always act in a manner that is in accordance with his professional commandments and universal moral values.

Personal integrity

Ideally, everyone in society should act according to an approved code of behaviour. In practice, uprightness is contaminated by social and professional socialisation. The interpretation of uprightness or other human values is influenced by many other factors such as the culture in which one is raised, the educational system where one learns to differentiate between right and wrong, and the system of monitoring and control including inside the family unit in which one is raised. Such a practice as disregarding consent is learned through professional socialisation and is passed on from experienced doctors to junior doctors. However, probity is a personal ethical characteristic which is not influenced by circumstances. For example, it is wrong to cheat your patients. It is wrong not to disclose relevant information to other professional colleagues in a grant or ethics approval application. It is wrong to commit scientific fraud.

Personal integrity is important in research and acts as a self-imposed limit on what is to be undertaken. Without it, there is a danger for the scientist to be tempted by the prospect of success that will lead to professional and social status or wealth. Professional desire to gain kudos, and general competitiveness, can lead scientists and doctors to commit fraud by falsifying data and being dishonest to grant committees. Sometimes experiments are faked, such as those in the recent stem cell research fraud in South Korea,[18] as a shortcut to proving a hypothesis that the scientist 'knows to be true'. The researcher may not even consciously consider that he/she is doing anything wrong. In some cases, patients and other people have been cheated in the process. The 1976 John Moore case highlighted below raised not only questions about the law, regulations and professional guidelines associated with medical research, but also ownership, consent and the integrity of some doctors.

Mr Moore first visited the University of California Los Angeles Medical Center in October 1976, shortly after learning that he had a rare type of hair-cell leukaemia. Blood and bone marrow contents were taken. His rare type of leukaemia was confirmed. A week later, the doctor in charge of Mr Moore's treatment recommended that his spleen be removed as part of the treatment of a life-threatening condition. Moore gave written consent. Before the operation the same doctor in charge made arrangements to obtain a portion of Mr Moore's spleen for study in a separate research unit but at the same time gave a written statement that 'these research activities were not intended to have...any relation to [Moore's] medical care'.[16] The patient's permission for the use of his spleen for research was not sought, nor was the research made known to him.

From November 1976 to September 1983 Mr Moore was required to visit the hospital for periodic check-ups. A sample of blood was taken during each visit. In fact, the doctor was conducting a series of researches on Mr Moore's cells and planned to benefit financially and competitively. The research relied on the doctor–patient relationship. During the course of the research, a patent was developed without Mr Moore's knowledge. His cells were used to extract a particular substance to treat patients with a similar condition.[16]

In the case above, the patient was misled by the doctor in charge. The living tissue obtained from Mr Moore was used for commercial purposes purely for the benefit of the doctor. It would seem that Mr Moore's case is not an isolated incident as in the United States concern about such unscrupulous practice is widespread. Wilmhurst cited a number of cases in the US at a seminar held at the British Medical Association in 1996, believing that 'in the US large-scale scientific dishonesty can be tolerated by peers and seniors'.[19]

In the UK, in the NHS and elsewhere the problem is that malpractices are not often reported by professional colleagues as whistle-blowing requires courage and integrity on the part of the whistle-blower, and is often perceived as unacceptable behaviour by peers and management. Many have suffered the consequences. For example, Betty Millar, an information technology manager in a health trust, lost her job in 1996 after she raised concerns about waste and irregularities in the purchase of supplies amounting to £240 000 in value.[20]

There are reports of many similar cases where people believed they could make a contribution by speaking out against bad practices and injustices. Public Concern at Work (a charity established in October 1993 to help see that employees raise and employers address concerns about malpractice in the workplace) defended three employees following disclosure of malpractices in the commercial sector.[21] In the NHS, Graham Pink lost his job as a night nurse having reported that the standards of elderly care in the ward in which he worked suffered from shortages of staff and that patients were badly treated.[22] An anaesthetist at the Bristol Royal Infirmary had to seek another job in another country after raising his concerns regarding the mortality rates of children who had undergone heart surgery at the Infirmary. The poor outcome of these children was confirmed by the inquiry which followed.[21]

In the past there has been a reluctance to recognise that scientific misconduct has been a problem in the UK, a similar ethos to that held in the US. Wilmshurst, in his article 'The code of silence' published in *The Lancet*, contends that 'those who should uphold the ethics of medicine and medical research tolerate and help to conceal dishonesty. As a result, the entitlement of the profession to regulate itself must be questioned.'[19] Generally, it appears that institutions such as the NHS were not greatly disposed to take action when they had information of possible irregularities. Now, 'after years of denying the existence of scientific misconduct in the UK, the establishment has admitted that there is some, as the General Medical Council has struck off several doctors who were reported for scientific misconduct by the Association of the British Pharmaceutical Industry.'[19]

There is an element of competitiveness in research. Some scientists are more driven by professional recognition and the desire to be first 'in the game'. The introduction of the oral poliomyelitis vaccine, referred to in Chapter 2, is such an example. It is a human frailty, which might also have been responsible for tempting the doctors in Moore's case.[16] More recently, the stem cell research fraud in South Korea mentioned previously serves to demonstrate the damage which can be done to individuals in the scientific world if one chooses to deviate from the moral path.[18]

During the last few years the public has raised doubts about the integrity of researchers. During the Isaacs Inquiry (referred to briefly in Chapter 1; *see also* Chapter 5), the integrity of the principal researcher in brain research was subject to question. The Isaacs Report stated that 'Most of the brains from coroners' cases in the 1980s and 1990s were initially held for entirely proper diagnostic investigation into the cause of death. A very much smaller number were retained specifically for research and teaching. The feature that unifies both these categories is that very few relatives were aware of the practice and I found no evidence that any were asked for their consent for later research or teaching use. In this way the requirements of the Human Tissue Act 1961 were consistently disregarded. It appears that the assumption was made that a signed post-mortem consent form also indicated agreement to organ and tissue retention.'[23] Her Majesty's Inspector of Anatomy raised 17 unanswered questions in the Isaacs Report about the joint research programme. These included:

- why were coroners not explicitly asked for their agreement to retention of brains for the research programme?
- why were ethics committees not explicitly informed about the joint research programme's plan to use brains from coroners' cases?
- why was the intention to collect brains from coroners' cases not made explicit in the applications to research funding bodies?
- why were there no references to coroners' cases in the 1988 application to the North West Regional Health Authority when the research team knew that 52 out of the 61 brains collected by the programme before that date had been retained from coroners' cases?
- why were in-patients in mental hospitals who had no relatives referred to in the following manner: 'often chronic in-patients don't have next-of-kin, in which case there is no difficulty', when the NHS guidance circular required consent from the hospital secretary/chief executive, who should have made their own investigations before agreeing to the post-mortem?

From these questions one suspects there was an intention to use deception in order to obtain consent from the research ethics committees and the funding bodies. Using deception in one's professional capacity is erroneous. According to Kant there is no justification on moral grounds for anyone to deliberately deceive others: 'A human action is morally good, not because it is done from immediate inclination, still less because it is done from self-interest, but because it is done for the sake of duty.'[24] The term 'duty' should be interpreted to mean that as human agents there is an obligation for us to act rationally and do what we ought. The 'ought' is a moral command necessitating one to act in accordance with law.[24]

The discussion on the code of ethics in medical research has set the boundary for case analysis in the next few chapters. In recent years there have been incidences similar to Mr Moore's case in the US,[16] where the law governing the use of human tissue for practice, teaching and research has been broken. In many situations ethical rules have been contravened and rules regarding human rights violated by the medical profession. The legal system appears to be powerless to protect the public interest and more and more members of the public are seeking justice against those who have committed serious professional misconduct.

References

1 Plato. *The Republic*. Lee D, tr. London: Penguin Books; 1955.
2 Green P. Letter from the president of the Royal Statistical Society to the Lord Chancellor regarding the use of statistical evidence in court cases. London: Royal Statistical Society; January 2002.
3 Studd H. GMC investigates cot-death expert over wrong sums. *The Times*, 12 June 2003: 14.
4 Kant I. *Groundwork of the Metaphysics of Morals*. Gregor M, tr. Cambridge: Cambridge University Press; 1991.
5 The Shipman Inquiry: 3rd and 4th Reports. London: The Stationery Office; 2003.
6 Boseley S. Obstetricians call for debate on ethics of euthanasia for very sick babies. *Guardian*; 6 November 2006; 8.
7 Department of Health. Good Doctors, Safer Patients: a report by the Chief Medical Officer. London: Central Office of Information; 2006.
8 Irvine D. Doctors in the UK: their new professionalism and its regulatory framework. *The Lancet*. 2001; **358:** 1807–10.
9 General Medical Council. *General Medical Practice*. 3rd ed. London: GMC; 2001.
10 Nuremberg Code: permissible medical experiments. Washington: US Government Printing Office; 1949: 181–2.
11 World Medical Association Declaration of Helsinki. Ethical principles for medical research involving human subjects [accessed Sept 2006]. Available from: www.wma.net/e/policy/b3.htm
12 The Belmont Report. Ethical Principles and Guidelines for the Protection of Human Subjects of Research. Washington, DC: US Government Printing Office; 1979.
13 Convention on Rights of the Child. [accessed Nov 2004] Available from: http://en.wikpedia.org/wiki/Convention_on_the_Rights_of_the_Child.
14 Human Rights Act 1998: Elizabeth II. Chapter 22. The Stationery Office; 1998.
15 Illich I. *Medical Nemesis: the expropriation of health*. London: Calder & Boyars Ltd; 1975.
16 Nuffield Council on Bioethics. Human Tissue: ethical and legal issues. London: NCB; 1995.
17 NHS Central Office for Research Ethics Committee (COREC). The use of human organs and tissue. An interim statement. London: Department of Health; 2003. © Crown copyright.
18 BBC News. Hwang apologises to South Koreans. [Accessed Nov 2006] Available from: http://news.bbc.co.uk/2/asia-pacific/4604464.stm.
19 Wilmhurst P. The code of silence. *Lancet*. 1997; **349:** 567–9.
20 Freedom to Care. Caring Services Network – Betty Millar's story. Surrey: The Whistle: 1977; 13.
21 Public Concern at Work. Case studies 1, 2 and 3. 2nd Annual Report. London: Public Concern at Work; 1996; 91–8.
22 Mathieson A. Code of conduct could put your job in danger. *Nursing Standard*. 1998; **12(28):** 9.

23 Department of Health. The Isaacs Report: the investigation of events that followed the death of Cyril Mark Isaacs. London: The Stationery Office; 2003.

24 Kant I, cited by Paton HJ. *The Moral Law*. London: Hutchinson & Co. Ltd; 1948.

25 Cheung P. Phenomenology of nursing [PhD dissertation]. Southampton: Univ. Southampton; 1992.

Chapter 4

Law, medical research and the public

Introduction

Medical education, practice and research are governed principally by several pieces of legislation developed during the 19th, 20th and 21st centuries. Religion and rules from the earlier centuries have had some control and influence over the study of anatomy and body dissection. From the 18th century onwards, the Houses of Parliament assumed the responsibility for the development of laws in medical studies, practice and research. As shown in Table 4.1, Acts passed by Parliament from 1752 to 2004 have had and continue to have a direct influence on the development of medical education and research.

Some Acts of Parliament, such as the Murder Act 1752, the Anatomy Act 1832 and the Human Tissue Act 2004, have had a turbulent passage in the Houses of Parliament, partly because of the sensitive nature of the subject matter, fear of public revolt, objections raised by the medical profession and most recently the active participation of many members of the public at various hearings of the Human Tissue Bill 2003. The public in the past had very little influence over how laws were made. They were the subjects for whom laws were made.

During the last few years, it has become clear that 'nationally, organ retention – with or without consent – had taken place.'[1] Members of the public in the UK (particularly in England) have strongly objected to those doctors and researchers directly and indirectly involved in hospital-based and coroners' post-mortems because of their non-compliance with the Human Tissue Act 1961, and have actively canvassed for a new law that will protect the rights of citizens in the future. It has been the first time in history that the voice of the public has been heard by Parliament, and the first time that politicians and the medical profession have failed to win over Parliament by persuasion. In view of this, it is important to give some attention in this chapter to examining the passage of these laws governing medicine and medical research, and the impact that they have had and will continue to have on society.

The study of anatomy is essentially a scientific subject prescribed for medical students during their undergraduate programme and in more specialised ways during postgraduate education. If you think about medical students you perhaps picture them being given a copy of *Gray's Anatomy* as they begin their long years of study. For example, in the last 30 years *Gray's Anatomy* has become a treasure house of stunning images, many of them made possible by imaging techniques pioneered in Britain. The pictures of detailed micro-anatomy are far removed from the old 'gross anatomy'.

The study of anatomy was long exemplified by Rembrandt's *Anatomy Lesson*, where we see dissection being performed in a 'theatre'. Today, the accustomed belief that the structure and functions of the human body can only be learned

Table 4.1 Dates and significant events in the development of human anatomy and dissection from the 3rd century BC to the 21st century

Date	People/Organisation	Significant Events
3rd century BC	Herophilus and Erasistratus	Discovered the brain was the centre of the nervous system. First anatomy school established
c. AD130–201	Galen	Experimental anatomy based on animal dissection
1163	Council of Tours edict	The dissection of human bodies prohibited
1283–1365	European countries	Legalisation of human dissection
1315	Mondino de Liuzzi	1st public dissection of executed criminals
Early 14th century	Pope Boniface VIII	Dissection forbidden
1506	James IV of Scotland	Royal patronage given to Edinburgh Surgeons and Barbers
1540	Henry VIII	Royal patronage given to barber-surgeons in England to dissect four hanged felons
1543	Andrea Vesalus, founder of modern anatomy	*De humani corporis fabrica* (anatomical dissections)
1556	Pope Paul VI	Papal ban on dissection lifted. Anatomy became key part of medical education
24 February 1562	Henry Machin (diarist)	First penal public dissection in England recorded
1628	William Harvey	Circulation of blood demonstrated
Mid 1600s	Charles II	Annual right to dissection of executed criminals increased in number from four to six
18th century	Philanthropists	Establishment of several London hospitals
18th century	The public	Frequent riots against the surgeons
1723–24	College of Barber-Surgeons	Attempt to obtain an Act of Parliament for securing executed bodies; Sheriff of London to deliver bodies of those not condemned to dissection to relatives
1745	William Cheseldon	A private anatomy school set up in Covent Garden
1763	William and John Hunter	Museum of anatomy set up in Soho, London; each student allowed one cadaver
1752	Houses of Parliament	The Murder Act 1752
1794	Town Council of Edinburgh	Act for requisition of bodies by the Royal College of Physicians and private anatomy schools
1811–12	Diary of a London Resurrectionist	Record of body snatchers' activities
1815	Houses of Parliament	Apothecaries Act 1815 – required licence to practise medicine, stipulating anatomy dissection. More private anatomy schools set up
1824–34	Universities	Medical schools in Birmingham, Leeds, Hull, Liverpool, Manchester, Sheffield and York established. Anatomy became formal study in medicine

1828–29	Burke and Hare	Committed murders to supply anatomy schools
1832	Houses of Parliament	Anatomy Act 1832 – provided legal acquisition of human bodies for dissection
1952	Houses of Parliament	Corneal Grafting Act 1952
1961	Houses of Parliament	Human Tissue Act 1961
2004	Houses of Parliament	Human Tissue Act 2004
2006	House of Commons	Draft Coroners Bill

from human dissection has been, and is being, challenged from within the medical profession. For example, the newest medical school in England – the Peninsula Medical School – has introduced a computer-imaging model for the teaching of anatomy instead of using cadavers. The school has abandoned 2300 years of tradition so that medical students do not engage in human dissection during their basic medical education. How competent the doctors who qualify from the Peninsula Medical School will be when compared with those trained by the traditional methods remains to be seen. A new trend has started in medical education and in the field of human anatomy; however, this new trend is not left unchallenged. The traditional medical degree consists of two years of academic work, including dissection, before a student meets a patient. Some medical practitioners are strongly opposed to the Peninsula model of teaching anatomy. This is based on the proposition that 'it is important for students to become accustomed to the concept and smells of death, and the dissection of a real specimen is the only way to gain a three-dimensional perspective of a human body.'[2]

Historical context

The development of the medical profession itself, and the use of human bodies for teaching, practice and research, have a long history. Anatomy has been an important part of the study of medicine for centuries. Herophilus and Erasistratus, acknowledged as 'the originators of dissecting', founded the first school of anatomy in Alexandria during the 3rd century BC.[2] Based on his anatomical dissection of 600 human corpses, Herophilus demonstrated that the brain was the centre of the nervous system.[3] We do not know for certain how those human corpses were obtained nor can we be certain when and how the discovery would have taken place without human dissection. Since the 3rd century BC, developments in the study of human anatomy have continued under many different social and political circumstances. Table 4.1 outlines some of the significant events from that time until the 21st century.

The Greek physician Galen has been acknowledged for his work on experimental physiology and he stressed the importance of anatomy in understanding the functioning of the body. It can be said that through Galen's work, human dissection was eventually legalised. It should be emphasised that during Galen's period, human dissection was prohibited and most of his dissections were carried out on animals. Galen's influence on the European view of medicine, including anatomy, has spanned well over 1000 years.[3,5]

The dissection of human bodies continued to be prohibited by religious authority under the Council of Tours edict, 1163.[4] In the 13th century, the realisation that human anatomy could only be taught by dissection of the human body resulted in its legalisation in several European countries between 1283 and 1365. 'Anatomia publica' – the public dissection of executed criminals – was subsequently introduced. Mondino de Liuzzi performed the first recorded public dissection of an executed criminal *circa* 1315.[6,7] This was contrary to the decree of Pope Boniface VIII earlier in the century, which forbid the dissection of human corpses for the study of anatomy.[8]

The founder of modern anatomy is considered to be Andreas Vesalius. Due to the papal ban Vesalius is thought to have worked in secrecy, visiting places of execution at night to perform dissection by torchlight.[9] His work on anatomical dissection was published in 1543 in *De Humani Corporis Fabrica*.[6] The publication of this illustrated book on the structure of the human body posed a serious challenge to religious authorities. He was accused of grave robbing and gibbeting. The Inquisition issued a death sentence upon him, which forced him to flee to Jerusalem.[4,9]

In Britain, dissection of human bodies remained proscribed until the 16th century. In 1506, James IV of Scotland gave royal patronage to the Edinburgh surgeons and barbers, which allowed them to dissect the 'bodies of certain executed criminals'.[10] In 1540, Henry VIII gave similar patronage to the Barber-Surgeons in England, giving them 'an annual right to [dissect] the bodies of four hanged felons'.[10] The permission was increased to six by Charles II. Diarist Henry Machin recorded one of the earliest penal dissections that took place in England on 24 February 1561.[11] Eventually, the papal ban on human dissection was lifted in 1556.[9] It is difficult to understand why Pope Paul VI lifted the ban; maybe he was influenced by his advisers who, in turn, were canvassed by influential anatomists. This would not be an unreasonable explanation, as even now canvassing takes place. Perhaps the religious hierarchy had begun to recognise that the study of human anatomy was an essential science and could contribute to the treatment of ill health. From then the empirical study of human anatomy became a key part of medical education.[2]

The lifting of prohibition on human dissection allowed further scientific discoveries, which challenged both accepted medical knowledge and religious ideas about the body. In 1628, William Harvey demonstrated the circulation of blood around the body.[6] Harvey's discovery dismissed Galen's four temperaments or humours,[3] and revealed that the body was basically a machine that could be repaired. Such an idea gave rise to the profession of the surgeon.[7]

Acts of Parliament governing the study of anatomy

In the following sections of this chapter, the relevant Acts of Parliament relating to the study of anatomy will be discussed. It is hoped that this will shed some light on the social issues involved and the position of the public throughout the centuries. Some Acts of Parliament have had a turbulent passage because of the sensitive nature of the subject matter, and in some cases the public reacted violently, believing that they were being disadvantaged by the medical profession and the politicians. During the passage of certain Acts during the 19th and 20th centuries, the public was in fact the subject of these Acts.

However, in 2003 the public took an active part in campaigning for change in a law that governed the use of the human body and human body parts for education and research.

The Murder Act 1752: the legalisation of human dissection

During the first half of the 18th century five major hospitals were founded in London. Most provincial towns had their own hospital by the end of the century, creating a number of teaching centres.[12,13] At this time the dissection of human corpses was restricted to the Royal College of Physicians and the Company of Barber-Surgeons, who were only allowed an annual allocation of 10 corpses between them.[14] This monopoly on human corpses for dissection made it virtually impossible for these new teaching centres to teach anatomy. The lack of bodies for dissection in some areas led to direct intervention from the local authority in order to ensure a sufficient supply. For example, in 1694 the town council in Edinburgh passed an Act enabling an anatomist to acquire bodies 'of such as may be found dead in the streets, and the bodies of such as die violent deaths...who shall have nobody to own them...' In addition, other bodies could be demanded: foundlings who had died after being weaned and after being put to school could be claimed unless their friends reimbursed the kirk treasurer whatever they had cost the town; the bodies of infants stifled at birth and unclaimed by any citizen; and the bodies of 'such as are *felo de se* [suicide]'.[11]

In 1723–24, the College of Barber-Surgeons attempted to instigate an Act of Parliament for securing executed bodies. On several occasions surgeons petitioned Parliament, complaining of the difficulties in securing corpses under the royal charter and requesting that guards should attend the hangings in order to control the crowds. The life of the surgeon was made even more difficult as obtaining corpses from hanging fairs was often riotous, as relatives and friends of the executed attempted to rescue the corpse. Battles often ensued. In order to prevent these disturbances, the Sheriff of London undertook to deliver those bodies not condemned to dissection to their friends or relatives for burial.[14]

In 1745, Surgeon-Anatomist William Cheseldon attempted to establish a Surgeons' Hall for the purpose of teaching anatomy by dissection; however, his attempt failed[13] as dissection of human corpses in London at that time was restricted to the Royal College of Physicians and the Company of Barber-Surgeons who were only allowed access to ten corpses between them each year. In 1746, William Hunter began teaching anatomy at a private school in Covent Garden, and in 1763, together with his brother John, he set up a museum of anatomy based in Soho.[7] Hunter was said to have taught anatomy in the 'Parisian manner', each student having access to an individual corpse .[10] This created an increased demand for corpses and caused further problems for the surgeons.

The need to quell the riots, furnish the surgeons' demands for more bodies and provide a punishment for and deterrence from committing murder resulted in the passing of the Murder Act in 1752: 'an Act for preventing the horrid crime of murder'.[14] The Act stipulated that, after execution, all murderers should be 'dissected and anatomised' (*sic*) or gibbeted in order to deny the individual a Christian burial.[11,15] The purpose of this penal dissection was more to do with the dishonour it would bring upon those who committed murder than the medical knowledge gained by the dissection of the body.[14] However, it did release more corpses for dissection, but only to the 'Hall of the Surgeons' Company'.[11] Having said that, surgeons did benefit financially, as the cost of obtaining bodies from the gallows reduced from £118.1s in the period between 1735–40 to £3.9s during the years 1750–55. Under the Murder Act, anyone caught attempting to rescue from the gallows those condemned to anatomisation risked seven years' transportation.[9] From 1752 dissection was seen, both legally and socially, as 'a fate worse than death'.[15]

The Apothecaries Act 1815 and the Anatomy Act 1832

An increase in the population between the 1750s and 1830s led to the need for more doctors[16,17] and the subsequent development of more medical schools. Between 1824 and 1834, medical schools that taught anatomy were established in Birmingham, Bristol, Leeds, Hull, Liverpool, Manchester, Newcastle, Sheffield and York; Sheffield also had a private school of anatomy.[5] The need for more bodies was exacerbated further by the introduction of the Apothecaries Act in 1815, instituting a professional self-regulation system whereby no one could practise medicine without a licence. The prerequisite for a licence to practise was that individuals had to attend specific courses, including anatomy.[13,16] Consequently there was a proliferation of private anatomy schools, and by 1832 there were 17 such establishments in London alone.[17]

The demand for human cadavers for the teaching of anatomy could not be met by the allowance stipulated under the 1752 Murder Act and, as a result, using present-day terminology, an internal competitive market was created. Private anatomy schools did not have the legal status to practise anatomical dissection and had no legal access to human cadavers.[17] The human body became a commodity. In Scotland, it was possible to pay fees in corpses rather than cash and grave robbing seemed to be an easy source of obtaining human bodies for dissection. Apprentice surgeons apparently indulged in this activity as, in 1721, a clause was put into their contract that banned them from associating with the exhumation of human corpses.[10]

One can imagine that when the rules on the acquisition of bodies for the study of anatomy were relaxed, unscrupulous and opportunistic practices would result. It should be noted that during this period grave robbing was not illegal, as the dead body could not be owned and, therefore, could not be stolen. Only if the robbers were found guilty of stealing property from the grave or corpse were they punished, usually by whipping.[10] In fact, the issue of ownership of the body remains unresolved until the present time. However, the acquisition of bodies from graves specifically for dissection was illegal, as the law only authorised the dissection of criminals executed for murder, not other capital offences.[18] In 1785, of the 97 men hanged in the London area, only one had been convicted of murder.[18] The demand for bodies was outstripping the supply; in 1826, anatomy schools in London alone dissected 592 individuals.[10] 'As a result the "trade" of body snatching was developed to satisfy the medical schools' need to teach anatomy.'[18]

The Diary of a London Resurrectionist, 1811–1812 recorded the activities of a gang of body snatchers.[19] The gang obtained bodies from cemeteries or mortuaries and supplied them to named surgeons and anatomists in London. They also supplied corpses to Edinburgh. The corpses of both adults and children were taken, as well as fetuses. The diary stated that up to 19 bodies were stolen in a single night. If the bodies were too decomposed for dissection, the canine teeth were taken and sold.[19]

Clearly, the 1752 Murder Act could not satisfy the demand for the number of human cadavers required for anatomy teaching. In 1828, Sir Ashley Cooper stated, when giving evidence to a House of Commons select committee that there were 700 anatomy students in London at that time, but only 450 bodies were supplied annually. It was estimated that between four and 12 bodies were required for each of these students.[20] The 'resurrectionist trade' took advantage of the market forces and became the main suppliers of human bodies for the teaching of anatomy.

The acquisition of human corpses for the study of anatomy entered another league when William Burke and William Hare were found to have murdered innocent people, mainly the poor, to supply anatomy schools in Edinburgh. However, Edinburgh was not the only place where murders were taking place in order to satisfy the market demand for human corpses. In November 1831, the body of a teenage boy was offered to King's College, London, for dissection. The condition of the corpse was such that staff at the college suspected that the boy had been murdered. The police were informed and John Bishop, James May, James Shield and Thomas Williams were remanded in custody until an inquest had been held. The result of the inquest showed that the boy had not died from natural causes and these four men had been seen in a public house that was known to be a regular meeting place for body snatchers.

A search of Bishop's house produced articles of clothing which belonged to the dead boy and two other victims. Bishop, May and Williams were detained further, accused of murder and stood trial on 2 December 1831. All three men were found guilty of murder and sentenced to execution. On 4 December 1831, Bishop confessed to having murdered the two boys and one woman, and named Williams as the accomplice but stated that May was not involved. Bishop and Williams were hanged in front of a crowd of 30 000 and their dissected bodies were exhibited to the public.[21] It is thought that Bishop and Williams murdered 60 people during their activities as the 'London Burkers'.[22]

On 14 March 1828, the subject of anatomy science was brought to the attention of the House of Lords by the Marquis of Lansdowne, with a petition raised by 'a body of surgeons' and signed by its president, which expressed the surgical profession's concerns that they were placed in the position of 'total absence of means of procuring bodies for the purpose of dissection' and that the present legislation required 'persons engaging in that profession to go through a course of studies, in which the dissection of bodies formed a necessary ingredient'.[23] The surgeons were concerned because the profession was expanding and, due to the lack of human bodies for dissection, 'a considerable number of young students were compelled to pursue their studies in other countries, and particularly in France, where great facilities were afforded to them in procuring the necessary instruction'.[23]

The subject was subsequently raised in the House of Commons by the then Home Secretary, Robert Peel, on 21 April 1828. This time the petition was signed by the president of the council of the Royal College of Surgeons, Sir W Blizard, and council members such as John Abernethy and Sir Astley Cooper, as well as many other eminent members of the profession. Peel reiterated Lansdowne's support for the scientific study of anatomy which 'could not be learned by

models' and that 'the law required a man to possess a certain portion of information in his profession, and that they were liable to prosecution for professional ignorance.' The House was informed by Peel that 'he was afraid of public
discussion on the subject, when he recollected the prejudices which were found
to prevail, more particularly among the lower orders.'[23] It is no wonder that the
'lower orders' would react angrily to the matter raised by the House of
Commons, as the 1752 Murder Act targeted criminals. The reference to 'lower
orders' is no longer relevant in the 21st century as class discrimination has no
place in the UK and, more importantly, laws governing the medical profession
and the research communities affect the whole social spectrum.

In the light of history we can see that doctors had, and still have, a strong
influence on legislating change for the benefit of their profession, and politicians appear to have sympathy for their cause. It was upon pressure from the
Royal College of Physicians in Scotland that the town council in Edinburgh
passed their 1674 Act, the prime targets of which were the homeless, particularly young orphans, abandoned babies and those unfortunate individuals who
found life so hard they committed suicide.[11]

The discussion so far gives the impression that those in government at the
time appeared to hold the view that the state had a right to decide, for certain
categories of individuals, what happened to their bodies after death. For
example, during a session in the House of Commons in 1828, Sir Joseph Yorke
proposed that 'it would be proper to give up the bodies for dissection' of those
who committed suicide in London each year.[23] I suspect that families in the UK
would now meet such a proposition with strong protestation, as the proposal
was bizarre, aberrant and inhumane. Unfortunately, the attitude in the 19th
century appears to be relevant even today, as demonstrated in the Isaacs Report,
which describes how brains from the mentally ill were removed without the
consent of relatives.[24] The problem of the state having a say in the treatment
of the dead body was raised again by Paul Burstow, MP in a 2004 parliamentary session under the guise of presumed consent.[25]

The House of Commons in 1828 felt inclined to support the petition, as they
believed that the whole of society was indebted to the medical profession. A
select committee was appointed in April 1828 to 'inquire into the manner of
obtaining subjects for the schools of anatomy, and the state of the law affecting persons employed in obtaining or dissecting bodies.'[26]

In March 1829, the select committee reported, 'as the result of their enquiries,
that, as the law now stood, the science of anatomy must rapidly sink into decay;
as the difficulty of obtaining subjects was so great that the students were
themselves obliged to have recourse to the practice of exhumation, in order to
attain such a knowledge of anatomy as was necessary to render them capable of
practising on the human frame'.[27] Warburton argued that if 'some alteration were
not made in the law, the trade in human bodies, which it appeared led to the
commission of so many other crimes, could never be effectually put an end to'.[27]
Warburton said that in submitting the Bill to the House it was not his intention
'to impose any penalties or prohibitions: his wish was that legality should be
given, in certain cases, to practical anatomy. He proposed, therefore, that
anatomy should be considered lawful, if practised either in those cities or towns
which have universities or corporations having the power of conferring medical
preferment or degrees, or…hospitals established for the reception of 50 patients

at a time.'[27] He further moved that 'if no supply was to be derived by legal or authorised means … [then] it should be lawful for the overseers and managers of the poorhouses or workhouses, for the governors of prisons and of hospitals, to give up to any physician who may be a teacher of anatomy, for the purposes of dissection, the bodies of those persons who might not be claimed within a specified time by any friend or relative.'[27] As a result of such deliberations, it was said that 'if the project was adopted, it would be the means of exonerating hereafter a beneficent and humane profession from the possibility of being implicated in the charge of being confederates with either resurrection-men or a class of villains whose atrocities had so very recently been brought to light.'[27]

The recent atrocities referred to are the crimes committed by Burke and Hare and the involvement of the anatomist Robert Knox. The proposed Bill would exonerate anatomists such as Knox, as the study of anatomy would be legalised.

One can argue that the proposed Bill was inhumane, as it was inclined to treat the poor and the desperate as if they were of no social significance. They were seen as 'objects' to be given up to a noble and humane profession. It would seem that in the 19th century the ruling class had an advantage over the poor. In some ways, making dissection legal would protect the rich from exhumation by those who would be willing to commit this violation of decency. Many in the House of Commons were inclined to present justification for the proposed Bill by suggesting, for example, that:

> 'Besides, the poor themselves would be the parties most benefited by the measure; for the rich possessed the means of obtaining professional efficiency far beyond those within the reach of the poorer classes; upon whom, therefore, all improvements in medical science must have a more direct effect.'[28]

> 'No measure appeared to him so unobjectionable, as giving permission to the managers of hospitals to devote the bodies of such persons as had no relations to claim them, to the purposes of anatomy. …The poor went into the hospitals with the hope of being cured, and were regardless of the fate of their bodies after death.'[29]

By contrast, on 8 May 1829, Bransby Cooper presented a petition against the Anatomy Bill on behalf of the Royal College of Surgeons in regard to some clauses relating to licensing of anatomy schools.[30] During the debate in the House of Commons there were some objections raised. However, the second reading of the Bill was supported by a majority of 40, with eight against. The Anatomy Bill was committed on 15 May 1829 and the third reading took place on 19 May 1829.[31] It received its first reading in the House of Lords on 20 May 1829. The Lords perceived the subject 'of very great importance, but extremely unpopular out of doors'.[31] In response, *The Lancet*, dated 5 June 1829, objected to it, saying that it was a Bill:

> '… to prevent country surgeons from studying anatomy, to encourage the disinterment of the dead, to facilitate the exportation of dead bodies to Ireland, to promote the sale of dead bodies, and to inflict upon the bodies of the poor the same marks of ignominy and punishment as are branded upon the bodies of murderers.'[32]

At their sitting on 5 June 1829, the House of Lords moved that the proposed Bill be postponed because of objections raised. The Earl of Malmesbury objected 'to the principle of interfering with the bodies of persons who had not offended against the laws.'[33] The Earl of Haddington objected to the Bill even though 'subsequent to dissection...bodies would be decently buried.'[33] A strong objection was also raised by the Earl of Harwood, who said the government had 'no right to pursue people beyond the limits of the grave.'[34] The Archbishop of Canterbury suggested that '... by the next year, a measure might be introduced less offensive to the feelings of the community, and therefore less objectionable.'[35] The postponement was supported in order to avoid unnecessary public outcry against any proposed treatment of the poor. The Anatomy Bill was withdrawn.

Although the Bill had been dismissed by Parliament, the medical profession did not let the subject lie and the surgeons continued to petition both Houses of Parliament. The next we hear of the Bill is on 9 December 1831, when the Earl of Harrowby presented a petition from the 'Hunterian Society' to the House of Lords. The petitioners pointed out that the subject was first raised in 1828 and that attention ought to be given to it because 'as the law now stood, subjects could not be procured for anatomists without exposing the parties to prosecution for misdemeanors (*sic*), or prompting those parties to the commission of crimes' and 'that it was quite impossible for students, surgeons and others to attain expertness in, and the requisite qualifications for, their professions'.[36]

The Lord Chancellor felt it was his duty to point out that:

'... in the present excited state of the public mind, it would be as well to avoid all discussion on the subject, and that it would be especially wise to delay any legislative measure regarding it till that excitement had abated.'[37]

The public excitement referred to here is that of the exposé and execution of Bishop and Williams, the 'London Burkers'.

In light of the social unrest caused by body snatching, grave robbing and the anger against doctors, public opinion at the time was such that something had to be done to change the law regarding the provision of legally acquired corpses for the teaching of anatomy by dissection. On 15 December 1831, a second attempt was made to get the Bill through Parliament, 10 days after the hanging and dissecting of Bishop and Williams, the 'London Burkers'.[22]

During the House of Commons session on 15 December amendments to the 1828–29 Bill were put forward. Having considered the profession's objection to licensing, Henry Warburton suggested that it would 'be sufficient if inspectors were appointed by The Home Secretary'.[38] Anatomy schools were to be inspected. Warburton also suggested that the former Bill 'subjected the poor to considerable hardships, inasmuch as its operation was, in a great degree, confined to them'. He proposed the introduction of a clause 'which should be equally applicable to all classes in society'.[38]

The debate about various objections continued into 1832. Further petitions were raised by the Faculty of Physics in London, the Surgeons of Halifax and 288 students of St Bartholomew's Hospital.[39–41] However, there was no petition from the poor.[42] On 15 February 1832, a petition to the House of Commons from 'certain inhabitants of Blackburn, in Lancashire' asked the House to stop the 'Dead Body Bill'.[42] During the session on 27 February 1832, several amendments were suggested, including the following by Rigby Wason:[43]

- licensing of anatomy schools
- teachers of anatomy to have particular qualifications and to be licensed
- all bodies received for dissection to be registered; non-registry or false-registry to carry the penalty of a fine or imprisonment
- workhouses to keep a registry of bodies sent for dissection
- no body to be sent for dissection if 'certain' relatives objected
- any prosecutions to be brought to commence within six months of the incident
- executed murderers not to be dissected.

Further amendments were put forward to the House of Commons on 18 April. Warburton proposed that the Bill should authorise the 'parties having the lawful custody of bodies to dispose of them for the purpose of dissection, unless the deceased shall have expressed a desire to the contrary, either in writing or verbally before two witnesses'.[44]

Despite the fact that the medical profession had raised objections, and that most petitions presented to the House of Commons were against it,[45] the Bill progressed with some amendments. In particular:

- the appointment of (paid) Inspectors of Anatomy to oversee the distribution and legality of the corpses procured by the schools of anatomy[46]
- the legislation would be extended to include Ireland[47]
- the timing for contacting deceased relatives was increased from 24 hours to 48 hours after death.[48]

The main reason for supporting the Anatomy Regulatory Bill in the 19th century was that by legalising dissection, it would do away with 'burking' and enable the surgical profession to secure a sufficient number of bodies for dissection, without resorting to the help of 'resurrection men' who carried out their trade in defiance of the law. The Bill would also reduce the number of students leaving to study abroad – in other words, using current terminology, 'stop the brain drain'.

The principal objections raised in both Houses of Parliament during the 19th century were not too dissimilar to those arguments raised by members of the public and the families affected by the recent Alder Hey organ retention scandal (*see* below). During the four-year debate the principal objections were that the Bill was:

- inhumane – 'it was a Bill calculated to brutalise the human race' as it interfered with the bodies of people who had done nothing wrong[49,50]
- discriminatory – it targeted a disadvantaged group of people who needed medical care and social support. Individuals were put in a position from which they were unable to protest[51]
- unethical – it legalised the sale of dead bodies. It did not protect the disadvantaged and it interfered with the decent rites of sepulchre[52]
- insensitive – it did not take into consideration the feelings of the deceased's family.[53]

The trade in human corpses for anatomy schools led to the passing of the 1832 Anatomy Act,[54] which superseded the 80-year-old Murder Act of 1752. The new

Act provided the legal authority for anatomists to obtain human bodies for dissection from a range of sources, including the unclaimed bodies of the poor dying in hospital or the workhouse, rather than those of executed murderers. The punishment of dissection had been transferred from the murderer to the pauper.[22]

What can we learn from history? It is interesting to note that both past and present debates are remarkably similar. During the period between April 2001 and March 2004, while the Retained Organs Commission was attempting to deal with public concerns over the removal and retention of organs without public knowledge and consent, there was discussion by members of the medical profession and the public on the following subjects:

- the need for a continual supply of specimens for clinical audit, education and research
- the decline in post-mortem consents because of public objections and the lack of organs for transplantation
- the difficulties imposed on the medical profession if severe legal constraints were instituted in the new legal framework
- the need for students and doctors to have genuine body parts to learn from, as anatomy and pathology cannot be learned from models alone
- the right of the state over the deceased body
- the need for families to exhume their babies and children for multiple funerals
- the need to protect innocent people from events such as those in Liverpool (Alder Hey)
- the apparent bias of the government towards the medical profession.

The Corneal Grafting Act 1952

The Anatomy Act of 1832 did not allow the removal of human organs from the dead for purposes other than teaching and research. Future uses were then undreamed of and not really glimpsed for a hundred years. Advances in medicine and surgery, such as anaesthesia, insulin and penicillin, made healthcare a matter of much greater interest to the population as a whole. Because of these innovations a new area of medical advance followed the Second World War in the form of transplant surgery. The war had greatly encouraged progress in plastic surgery and wound healing; now a great new peacetime era of social progress had been ushered in with breathtaking advances, including the National Health Service, welfare provision and governmental interest in everyday life. Along with this came a new era in legislation.

In the 1950s a parliamentary bill was put forward for the purpose of corneal grafting. It took just six weeks and a day from its first reading in the House of Commons to attain royal assent on 26 June 1952.[55,56] The Corneal Grafting Act 1952 allowed individuals to bequeath their eyes for treatment purposes. It also allowed those 'in lawful possession of a body to permit the eyes to be taken, provided that there is no known objection from the dead person during his lifetime or from any relatives'.[55]

The Human Tissue Act 1961

In 1954, the first successful kidney transplant took place in Boston, USA. In the UK, the first live donor transplant was performed in 1960.[57] Such an advance in medical practice was fully supported by both Houses of Parliament. However, it was unlawful under existing legislation to use any parts, other than the corneas, for treatment purposes. To enable the medical profession to accomplish further progress in transplant surgery, a new law was necessary. In December 1960, Enoch Powell, the then Health Minister, presented the Human Tissue Bill to Parliament. The Bill proposed:

> '... to make provision with respect to the use of parts of bodies of deceased persons for therapeutic purposes and purposes of medical education and research and with respect to the circumstances in which post-mortem examinations may be carried out; and to permit the cremation of bodies removed for anatomical examination.'[58]

The Human Tissue Bill passed through Parliament in seven months and attained royal assent on 27 July 1961.[59] It was accompanied by a change in public perception regarding the acceptance of organ donation for transplant surgery and a willingness to bequeath one's body for medical research. These were pioneering days and there was optimism that lives would be saved. The Act was also coupled with a big publicity campaign encouraging donors to come forward,[60] whereas the Corneal Grafting Act 1952 was introduced under less open circumstances. The following was recorded in one of the parliamentary debates:

> '...for heaven's sake, do not raise this matter. Corneal grafting is going on, but the moment we give it any publicity there will be religious objections and the whole matter may come to an end. So please leave it alone.'[61]

Forty-five years on the legacy of secrecy, such as we have just seen in Hansard, is still with us and once again we are looking for openness in the new legislation on the use of human tissue.

The Anatomy Act 1984

The Anatomy Act 1984 'enables people to bequeath their bodies for anatomical examination by dissection for teaching, studying or research purposes'.[62] It differs from the Human Tissue Act 1961 in that:

> '... a request from an adult that his/her body should be used after death for anatomical examination must be made in writing, or exceptionally may be made orally in the presence of two witnesses during the person's final illness.'[62]

The 1984 Act also included some of the amendments put forward by Members of Parliament in their 19th-century debates on the study of anatomical science, such as:

- keeping full records of all anatomical specimens
- a bequeathed body must be disposed of by burial or cremation within three years of death
- Her Majesty's Inspector of Anatomy was to provide 'a central focus for information and administration throughout Great Britain', with the exception of the Isle of Man, the Channel Islands and Northern Ireland.[62]

The Anatomy Act 1984 repealed and replaced the Anatomy Act 1832.

The Human Tissue Act 2004

Following the disclosure of widespread illegal practice in organ removal and retention in England and Wales and throughout the rest of the UK, members of the public demanded a change in the law and have campaigned earnestly during the past few years.

On Wednesday 26 November 2003 the Queen's Speech confirmed that the government would introduce a new Human Tissue Bill[63] during the parliamentary session 2003–2004. The new Human Tissue Bill was published on 3 December 2003. The Bill arose from the public concerns highlighted in the Kennedy and Redfern Inquiries at the Bristol Royal Infirmary and the Royal Liverpool Children's Hospital (Alder Hey) that organs and tissue from children who had died had often been removed, stored and used without proper consent. When the new Bill was launched in December 2003, the then Secretary of State for Health, Dr John Reid, reiterated the public concerns by stating that the Bill will:

- 'Ensure that no human body parts, organs or tissues will be taken without the consent of relatives or patients. Once coroners' enquiries have concluded then organs and tissues taken will come under the authority of the Bill
- prevent a recurrence of the distress caused by retention of tissue and organs without proper consent by providing safeguards and penalties
- help improve public confidence so that people will be more willing to agree to valuable uses of tissue and organs like research and transplantation
- improve professional confidence so that proper authorised supplies of tissue for research, education and transplantation can be maintained and improved...'[64]

The new Human Tissue Bill was enacted in 2004. It is in three parts.

Part 1 deals with the removal of human material for schedule purposes with appropriate consent. The purposes requiring consent are: 'anatomical examination; determining the cause of death; establishing after a person's death the efficacy of any drug or other treatment administered to him; obtaining scientific or medical information about a living or deceased person which may be relevant to any other person, including a future person; public display; research in connection with disorders, or the functioning, of the human body and transplantation.'[65] Consent also applies to other activities such as 'clinical audit; education or training relating to human health; performance assessment; public health monitoring and quality assurance.'[65] Part 1 of the Act makes it an offence to carry out regulated activities without appropriate consent. It makes it unlawful to use bodies of human material, once donated, for purposes other than those set out, and establishes penalties. In terms of penalties, if a person is found guilty of using donated material for a purpose which is not a qualifying purpose or storing donated material for purposes other than the ones specified, then the person is liable:

'... on summary conviction, to a fine not exceeding the statutory maximum; on conviction on indictment

(i) to imprisonment for a term not exceeding three years, or
(ii) to a fine, or
(iii) to both.'[65]

Part 2 deals with the regulation of activities involving human tissue between living persons and prohibits commercial dealing in human material. It also sets out the remit of the Human Tissue Authority, licensing requirement and regulations. Penalties for those who are in breach of the licence requirement are set out in this part of the Act and are exactly the same as specified above.

Part 3 deals with various matters such as the power of the Human Tissue Authority to assist other public authorities for the purpose given to the Authority. The section in Part 3 of the Act that deals with human preservation for transplantation gives authority to the person having the control and management of a hospital, nursing home or other institution 'to take steps for the purposes of preserving the part for use for transplantation, and to retain the body for that purpose.'[65] Such authority 'ceases to apply once it has been established that consent making removal of the part for transplantation lawful has not been, and will not be, given.'[65] The Act also specifies that it is unlawful to make use of surplus tissue without consent including the non-consensual analysis of DNA.[65]

The new Human Tissue Act 2004 to some extent will provide reassurance that families will be protected in the future. However, one cannot determine the impact of the Act until it has been enacted and translated into practice. Its effectiveness will depend on the commitment of the health professionals to adhere to the law and internal policing mechanisms within each health trust. The management of each health trust will need to ensure that the Act is fully understood by those who are directly involved. Internal disciplinary mechanisms must be in place to manage those who flout the law.

The new Human Tissue Act 2004 repeals and replaces the Human Tissue Act 1961, the Anatomy Act 1984 and the Human Transplantation Act 1989 (this act regulates live organ transplants and commercial dealings in organs for transplantation removed from either living or dead people) as they relate to England and Wales. It also repeals and replaces the Human Tissue Act (Northern Ireland) 1962, the Human Transplants (Northern Ireland) Order 1989 and the Anatomy (Northern Ireland) Order 1992.

Public perceptions and law reforms

The 1752 Murder Act and the Anatomy Act of 1832 might have been seen by the public, particularly those who were poor, as working against them. They felt, expressed in present-day terms, that their rights as individuals had been usurped. In 1832, when referring to the Anatomy Bill, it was said: 'It placed individuals who died in hospitals on a footing with murderers for the bodies of both were to be given up to dissection.'[66] It should be noted that during the 19th century there were no social services, so the poor had to rely on philanthropists. Those who were poor and sick were accommodated in the poorhouses and workhouses provided by the do-gooders. Prior to 1834, the system of so-called poor relief was available without having to enter a workhouse. The 1834 Poor Law Amendment Act made entering a workhouse obligatory for able-bodied individuals requiring poor relief.[12]

However, the supply of bodies for dissection from the workhouse was secured by the fact that by 1832 the majority of paupers in the workhouse were sick and the mortality was high.[12,22] Most of the dead would be given up for dissection. Some would be protected from dissection after death because of their insurance – a 'penny policy' undertaken by them before entering a workhouse. Penny policies were burial insurances that most families would take out and contribute to weekly for all members of the family. Families who did not or could not take out such insurance risked the humiliation of 'a pauper's funeral' or dissection.[22]

The 1752 Murder Act was feared by condemned murderers, who would spend their last days attempting to secure a decent burial by contacting friends and relatives, requesting that they attend the hanging and take care of their body afterwards, thus avoiding dissection. Relatives would travel to London from as far as Carlisle, Lancashire and Lincoln, making substantial sacrifices in order to protect their own from surgeons taking possession of the corpse and to ensure a Christian burial; they would even guard the grave. Riots against the surgeons and their representatives were commonplace during the 18th and 19th centuries, particularly after hanging fairs.[14]

Around the same time as the Anatomy Bill was being discussed, the country was plagued by a cholera epidemic. The first case was recorded in Sunderland on 19 October 1831. The epidemic spread quickly and reached its height by June 1832. The Cholera Riots coincided with the passage of the Anatomy Act in 1832 and marked a definite turning point in public reaction to the way the poor were treated after death. The Liverpool Cholera Riots started on 29 May in response to a woman being taken into hospital. The violence was directed at the doctor who had ordered her removal to hospital, accusing him of 'burking' and 'murder'. It was estimated that 1000 rioters were involved. Further public unrest took place during the subsequent 10 days with similar accusations against the medical profession. The main cause of the Liverpool riots was the fear of body snatching.[67]

In 1999, the protest against the removal and retention of children's organs and body parts took on a more sophisticated form. The families and friends of the deceased children lobbied MPs and voluntary organisations with good effect, leading to inquiries being set up by the government.

The historical evidence presented here poses a number of fundamental issues from the public point of view. For example:

- was the introduction of various Acts concerned first and foremost with the notion of 'public good'?
- can the idea of 'public good' be sustained when the Hansard records are carefully examined?
- were the Murder Act 1752 and the Anatomy Act 1832 passed primarily for the benefit of the public?
- did these Acts have regard for the humanity of those who were seen to be socially marginalised, such as the poor and the criminals?
- how far was the public aware of the circumstances in which these Acts and their 20th-century successors were introduced?
- did the Human Tissue Act 1961 provide a sound framework for professional practice?
- to what extent did past legislation contribute to the unsatisfactory events of the last few decades?

We can conclude that Acts of Parliament governing medicine and medical research have brought hurt and suffering to many members of the public and some members of the medical profession. In this view, bad law led to individual flexible interpretation and the recognition of useful loopholes. For Martin Luther King, 'A just law is a man-made code which squares with the moral law or the law of God. An unjust law is a code that is out of harmony with the moral law.'[68] St Thomas Aquinas said: 'An unjust law is a human law that is not rooted in eternal and natural law. Any law that uplifts human responsibility is just. Any law that degrades human personality is unjust.'[69] Both religious leaders recognised a basic morality (which for them personally was God's law), which they plainly believed was synonymous with the human morality that all people seeking good would aim at.

References

1 Department of Health. Human bodies, human choices –the law on human organs and tissue in England and Wales. A consultation report. London: Department of Health Publications; 2002.

2 Le Bruxelles S. Medical school consigns cadavers to history. *The Times*, 9 Sept 2002; 3.

3 Garrison FH. *History of Medicine*. Philadelphia: Saunders; 1929; **103**: 112–17.

4 Lynch J. Contexts-science-biology-anatomy [accessed October 2002]. Available from: www.english.upenn.edu/%7Ejlynch/Frank/Contexts/anatomy.html.

5 Holmes RL. *The Melancholy of Anatomy*. Leeds: Leeds Univ. Press; 1967: 2.

6 Ellis P. Organ retention: balancing the needs of ethical research and respect for the dead [accessed Oct 2002]. Available from: www.lambchambers.co.uk/art5.htm.

7 The anatomists: the birth of medical anatomy [accessed Oct 2002]. Available from: www.channel4.com/science/microsites/A/anatomists/medicine2.html.

8 Cunningham A. *The Anatomical Renaissance*. Vermont: Scolar Press; 1997: 208.

9 Silverberg R. Reflections: burning science at the stake. Azimov's science fiction [accessed October 2002]. Available from: www.asimovs.com/_issue_0210/ref.shtml.

10 Johnson DR. Introductory anatomy [accessed October 2002]. Available from: www.leeds.ac.uk/chb/lectures/anatomy1.html.

11 Sawday J. *The Body Emblazoned*. London: Routledge; 1996: 60.

12 Lawrence C. *Medicine in the Making of Modern Britain,1700–1920*. London: Routledge; 1994: 20.

13 Cartwright FF. *A Social History of Medicine*. London: Longman; 1977: 48.

14 Linebaugh P. The Tyburn riot against the surgeons. In: D Hay *et al.*, editors. *Albion's Fatal Tree: crime and society in eighteenth-century England*. London: Penguin Books; 1975: 65–117; 79.

15 Richardson RA. Potted history of specimen taking. *Lancet*. 2000; **355**: 935–6.

16 Bynum WF. *Science and the Practice of Medicine in the Nineteenth Century*. Cambridge: Cambridge Univ. Press; 1994: 63.

17 Desmond A. *The Politics of Evolution*. Chicago, IL: Univ. of Chicago Press; 1989: 154.

18 Richardson S. Crime and punishment [accessed October 2002]. Available from: www.warwick.ac.uk/fac/arts/tecaching/courses/gender/crime.htm.

19 Boulton JP. The diary of a London Resurrectionist, 1811–1812 [accessed October 2002]. Available from: www.staff.ncl.ac.uk/j.p.boulton/deathtexts/naplesdiary.htm.

20 Kendall M. Anatomy teaching in Bristol [accessed October 2002]. Available from: http://d-mis-web.ana.bris.ac.uk/mark/anatomy_teaching_in_bristol.htm.

21 Pelham C. The Newgate calendar: John Bishop and Thomas Williams [accessed October 2002]. Available from: www.exclassic.org/newgate/ng609.htm.

22 Richardson R. 'Trading assassins' and the licensing of anatomy. In: R French, A Wear, editors. *British Medicine in an Age of Reform*. London: Routledge; 1991: 77.

23 Great Britain. House of Commons. Hansard. Official Report 1828; 18: 1136–7, 1612–13.

24 Department of Health. The Isaacs Report: the investigation of events that followed the death of Cyril Mark Isaacs. London: The Stationery Office; 2003.

25 Great Britain. House of Commons. Hansard. Official Report 2004; 416: 1010.

26 Ibid. 1828; 19: 15.

27 Ibid. 1889; 20: 998.

28 Ibid. 1829; 20:1004.

29 Ibid. 1829; 20: 1003.

30 Ibid. 1829; 21: 1167.

31 Ibid. 1829; 21: 1394–5, 1488–9.

32 Mr Wakley's petition. *Lancet*. 1828–29: **2**; 306.

33 Great Britain. House of Commons. Hansard. Official Report 1829; 21: 1474.

34 Ibid. 1829; 21: 1746–8.

35 Ibid. 1829; 21: 1746–8.

36 Ibid. 1831–32; 9: 132–3.

37 Ibid. 1831–32; 9: 133.

38 Ibid. 1831–32; 9: 300.

39 Ibid. 1831–32; 9: 1148.

40 Ibid. 1832; 9: 1183–5.

41 Ibid. 1832; 9: 1.

42 Ibid. 1832; 9: 1185.

43 Ibid. 1832; 10: 835–6.

44 Ibid. 1832; 12: 664.

45 Ibid. 1832; 12: 666.

46 Ibid. 1831–32; 9: 300.

47 Ibid. 1832; 12: 313.

48 Ibid. 1832; 12: 667.

49 Ibid. 1832; 12: 320.

50 Ibid. 1829; 21: 1747.

51 Ibid. 1829; 21: 1749.

52 Ibid. 1832; 13: 823–4.

53 Ibid. 1832; 13: 1086.

54 Edwards OD. *Burke and Hare*. Edinburgh: Polygon Books; 1980: 274.

55 Great Britain. House of Commons. Hansard. Official Report 1951–52; 502: 1445–7.

56 Ibid. 1951–52; 502: 2486.

57 NHS UK Transplant. Transplant milestones [accessed October 2002]. Available from: www.uktransplant.org.uk/about_transplantation_milestones/tranplantation. milestones.htm.

58 Great Britain. House of Commons. Hansard. Official Report 1960–61; 613: 1454.

59 Ibid. 1960–61; 644: 672.

60 Ibid. 1960–61; 632: 1240.

61 Ibid. 1960–61; 632: 1240.

62 Department of Health. Human Bodies, Human Choices: the law on human organs and tissue in England and Wales. A consultation report. London: Department of Health Publications; 2002. p. 21.

63 Great Britain. House of Commons. Human Tissue Bill 2003. London: The Stationery Office Ltd; 2003.

64 Department of Health. Reid makes consent cornerstone in new Human Tissue Bill. Press Release 2003/0493. London: Department of Health.

65 Human Tissue Act 2004. Elizabeth II. Chapter 30. London: The Stationery Office; 2004: 6–8.

66 Great Britain. House of Commons. Hansard. Official Report 1832; 12: 897.
67 Gill G. Fear and frustration: the Liverpool Cholera Riot of 1832. *Lancet.* 2001; **358**: 233–7.
68 Carson C. (ed.) *The Autobiography of Martin Luther-King, Jr.* London: Little, Brown & Co. Ltd; 1999.
69 Aquinas ST. *A Collection of Critical Essays.* London: Macmillan; 1969: 340–80.

Chapter 5

Non-compliance with the Human Tissue Act 1961 and its consequences

The Human Tissue Act 1961: not well understood

The Human Tissue Act 1961 was a key piece of legislation that the medical profession was required to follow. It was an Act of Parliament and failure to comply in any sense would constitute in principle a criminal act. In which case, individuals who disobeyed would be subject to penal punishment. The Act remained on the statute book for 43 years as it was believed that the law was being complied with by the medical profession, and there was no reason to think otherwise.

During the initial disclosure in 1995 of the unusually high mortality rate following paediatric cardiac surgery at Bristol Royal Infirmary, one of the parents discovered that her daughter's heart had been removed and retained at a post-mortem examination without her knowledge. It was at this point that members of the public began to realise that the law could have been broken by doctors and this illegal practice had been going on for many years without anyone's knowledge. Later, it was found that a similar practice had also taken place at the Royal Liverpool Children's Hospital (Alder Hey).

In fact, the practice of organ removal and retention started many years before any Acts of Parliament were passed, following the Anatomy Act 1832. A heart collection was established in 1948 by Dr (later Professor) John Hay and continued to grow over the years. Hearts were collected usually without parental knowledge. The collection was situated at the Institute of Child Health at Alder Hey Hospital. Most professionals across society are driven by the desire, sometimes without reflection, to do their best for their clients. Doctors are no different, but they should not underestimate the intelligence of those whom they serve. As Alder Hey showed, doctors cannot safely assume that the trust of the public is so great that they will not object to being deceived, even when the intention is good. *The Times*, in its obituary of Professor Hay, pointed out that:

> 'When Professor John Hay was appointed in 1939 as physician to the Royal Liverpool Children's Hospital, there was little that could be done for babies born with malformed hearts. He was determined after the war to find better ways of investigating and treating such unfortunate babies, who often died very quickly.'[1]

Professor Hay pioneered the use of cardiac catheterisation, which allowed him to investigate heart defects with accuracy. However, the technique alone could not save the babies and many still succumbed. He decided that the 'failures' should be studied, and therefore in 1948 he began a collection of hearts taken from babies at post-mortem. The collection was to play a leading role in improving cardiac services for children.[1] Professor Hay's obituary is a lesson in itself, in that, a totally committed doctor who saved many lives during his career can still become associated with a scandal and have his reputation tarnished by an 'apparently errant pathologist – van Velzen'.[1] Even so, it is all too easy to apportion blame to one particular individual, even if he is 'an errant pathologist'.

The problem is systemic. It should be noted that although there was no legislation governing post-mortem examination at the time when the Alder Hey heart collection began, there could have been awareness of the historical and legal context of human dissection and the consequences of following the same path; for example, with regard to the anatomy teachers in earlier centuries who were equated with resurrection men or body snatchers (*see* Chapter 4). Even if doctors who collected human organs did not take into account previous sensitive issues concerning body dissection, they should not have overlooked the implications of the Corneal Grafting Act 1952 and the subsequent Human Tissue Act 1961. From 1952 onwards, in the light of legislation, doctors at Alder Hey failed to give appropriate attention to the legal aspects of obtaining and using organs and body parts for treatment, education and research. They may have believed they should act outside the law in the interest of medical science. By October 2000, there were more than 2000 hearts in the collection. Without public protest in Liverpool, the collection would have continued to grow, with the doctors conducting their work in the belief that the public would continue to acquiesce.

One can appreciate the need for a change in the Human Tissue Act 1961, and the public in Liverpool campaigned for such a change. The Act was repealed and replaced by the Human Tissue Act 2004, which was described in the last chapter.

Having studied the appropriate legislation and having had first-hand experience of working with families over a range of issues relating to non-compliance of the Human Tissue Act 1961, the author has a better understanding of the reason why the Act was ignored or disregarded by practitioners. One of the reasons might be that the law was unclear, particularly regarding consent and the process by which consent was sought. Section 1, subsection 2 of the Act states that:

'Without prejudice to the foregoing subsection, the person lawfully in possession of the body of a deceased person may authorise the removal of any part from the body for use for the said purposes [therapeutic, education or research as stated in subsection 1] if, having made such reasonable enquiry as may be practicable, he has no reason to believe:
(i)   that the deceased had expressed an objection to his body being so dealt with after his death, and had not withdrawn it; or
(ii) that the surviving spouse or any surviving relative of the deceased objects to the body being so dealt with.'[2]

There are a number of ambiguities in the Act. For example, the concept of 'the person in lawful possession of the body of the deceased person may authorise the removal of any part from the body...' is unclear. It could mean the hospital doctor in charge; it could also be the coroner if the death was so reported. The safeguard for the public is that the person in lawful possession of the body must be in no doubt that the surviving spouse does not object to such a procedure. The legal status of the body is subject to further deliberations in Chapter

7, as one could argue that the person who organises the funeral has the ultimate authority.

The Act permits the use of organs and tissue to be used for therapeutic purposes, including transplantation. However, the consent of the relatives was given legal standing in the Human Tissue Act 1961. Section 1(2) makes it clear that the objections of relatives should be recognised and that tissues and organs should not be used for medical purposes when the relatives object.[3] It will become clear later in this chapter that in most circumstances throughout the UK, consent was not sought in the manner that was required of the doctor by law. It will also become clear that coroners in most cases have disobeyed the law prescribed for their practice.

One suspects there is little room in the undergraduate curriculum for supplementary subjects, such as knowledge of the law, however important they might seem. For the generalists in medicine, the value of having knowledge of the law may not have immediate relevance until they are faced with a particular situation. Unless one makes a special study of these laws, one would not know the significance of the content in each Act. The other problem is that the Acts are normally drafted in legal jargon and are not accessible in language terms to clinicians and members of the public.

It would appear from the events in Bristol and Liverpool that the Human Tissue Act 1961 was either misinterpreted or poorly understood by the medical profession. Written evidence submitted by a representative of the Royal College of Physicians of London to the Chief Medical Officer's Summit held in London, would seem to suggest that some doctors were aware of the legal rights of the relatives when consent was sought for organs to be retained following post-mortem examination, but for a variety of reasons chose not to follow the letter of the law. The statement from the Royal College of Physicians in London states that:

> 'It is true that specific consent for retention of organs and tissues was not usually sought. This was not because of an intention to deceive or conceal the purpose, but because it was assumed that acceptance of such actions was implicit in the consent given to the process of autopsy… It is also regrettable that there have been implications that such storage of organs and tissues has been thoughtless, cavalier and macabre.'[3]

During the Kennedy Inquiry in Bristol, the issue of hospital post-mortems was examined. A consultant pathologist to the Home Office, Professor Michael Alan Green, gave evidence to the inquiry team and he also talked about the way he was taught as a medical student to obtain consent from relatives for an autopsy. He also charted the changes in attitude, as he saw them, from the time that the Human Tissue Act 1961 was passed. He told the Inquiry:

> '…in the past, when obtaining consent to hospital post-mortems, the prevailing culture was not to go into details with the family of the deceased about precisely what was involved in a post-mortem.'[4]

> 'I qualified in 1960. The Human Tissue Act was passed in 1961. My generation was, therefore, taught by those who had always themselves been taught that there was no property in a dead body, and the general lesson that was drilled into me as a medical student was: be courteous,

be polite, explain that you are asking for permission for this autopsy because it will help others, both in learning and in the treatment of disease, but do not go into any more detail; it will upset the relatives and they might refuse consent. This was the attitude on which my generation was brought up.[4]

'Even when the notion of consent to a hospital post-mortem became more widespread in the medical profession, parents were still given few details either of what a hospital post-mortem actually involved or about the possibility or likelihood of the retention of human material after the hospital post-mortem. Parents were not told, or at least did not understand, that they would not be burying all of their child.[4]

'The Human Tissue Act was passed in 1961. At first it made little difference. I think everybody, both hospital management and clinicians, said: "But we are doing all this anyway. We have a consent form which we always have witnessed", and in those days there were no such things as bereavement counselling officers. It was usually the senior house officer or the registrar who saw the relatives and got permission, and you simply had a bald consent form which said: "I, being [the wife, husband, etc] of...hereby agree to an autopsy being carried out. I understand this will help advance medical knowledge", or words to that effect... There was nothing organ specific and equally, there was no option of a limited or restricted post-mortem...'[4]

The key message here is that had the medical profession chosen a more appropriate way of obtaining informed consent before the 1961 Act and had it followed the letter of the law after 1961, much unnecessary suffering experienced by the public would have been avoided.

Reference has been made above to Professor John Hay's heart collection. The specimens of heart were collected without consent as it was assumed that the public would not object. The prevailing medical ethos at the time would have been passed on to many junior doctors through the process of professionalisation, i.e. 'sitting by Nelly'. Also, it was not usual for junior doctors to question their experienced consultants or doctors in academic positions. The process of professionalisation continues, albeit inappropriately as has been shown, through generations of doctors.

Another contributory factor was that doctors wanted to protect relatives from knowing what was involved in post-mortem examination as they believed the public would be upset by the more intimate details. They have been proved wrong in this regard. However, the attitude of paternalism still exists in the health service as one often hears clinicians saying they cannot really tell the patient or his family because (the clinicians think) they don't want to know the diagnosis and prognosis.

What then are the consequences of not knowing about legislation governing one's professional activities? Is it advantageous for the doctors to be content with the knowledge passed on by their seniors, who have neither studied the Acts of Parliament governing their work nor questioned their accustomed practice? Are members of the public being disadvantaged as a result of the doctors' behaviour?

Organ retention in context

Organ retention in children

Bristol Royal Infirmary Inquiry

The paediatric cardiac service at Bristol became the subject of scrutiny in 1995 as the mortality rate was shown to be much higher than for other cardiac centres in the country. Bristol was one of the nine supra-regional centres funded through the Department of Health. Bristol Royal Infirmary was selected to develop a special neonatal and infant cardiac surgery service for children under one year of age for the South West, including Wales. Subsequently, three doctors, Dr Roylance, Mr Wisheart and Mr Dhasmana, were investigated by the General Medical Council.

The media played a significant role in some of the events leading up to the Bristol Royal Infirmary Inquiry. On 27 March 1996, the television programme *Dispatches* examined paediatric cardiac surgical services in Bristol. One of the parents, Mrs HR, whose daughter died in 1992 after open-heart surgery, watched the programme. She was prompted to contact the United Bristol Hospital Trust about the care of her daughter and made arrangements to review her daughter's medical notes. The mother knew that a post-mortem examination had been carried out on her daughter, having been told there would need to be a post-mortem because her daughter died in theatre. Mrs HR discovered in the medical notes that her daughter's heart had been removed and retained at post-mortem examination. She visited the hospital and viewed the heart. She then asked the pathologist present at the viewing: 'Who had the responsibility of informing parents about the issue of retaining human material?'[4]

In the light of Mrs HR's discovery, a small number of parents made enquiries directly to a paediatric pathologist at Bristol between 1996 and 1998. The hospital decided to 'await contact initiated by parents, recognising that some parents would find a direct approach from the hospital both unwelcome and distressing.'[4] In the meantime, a parent action group called the Bristol Heart Children Action Group was formed and its members met the then Secretary for Health, Frank Dobson, MP.

In June 1998, Frank Dobson announced the establishment of an inquiry 'into the management of the care of children receiving complex cardiac surgery at the Bristol Royal Infirmary between 1984 and 1995 and relevant related issues; to make findings as to the adequacy of the services provided; to establish what action was taken both within and outside the hospital to deal with concerns raised about the surgery; and to identify any failure to take appropriate action promptly.'[5] Professor Sir Ian Kennedy was appointed as chairman. Thus at Bristol there was a convergence of organ retention issues with wider treatment and operational problems. The final report[5] was published on 18 July 2001.

Although the central focus of the inquiry into the Bristol Royal Infirmary was concerned primarily with the high mortality rate of children after open-heart surgery, because of Mrs RH's discovery, aspects of post-mortem examination and the practice of removal and retention of children's organs were also investigated.[5] The interim report[4] had by and large focused on removal and retention of human material.

During the inquiry evidence was received from 577 witnesses, including 238 parents. Evidence specific to the national context of both coroners' post-mortems and hospital post-mortems was received from clinicians, pathologists, the Coroners' Society, the Coroner for Avon, the Home Office, the Royal Colleges of Pathologists and of Physicians, and from Bristol health trusts. The inquiry also received 900 000 pages of documents, including the medical records of 1800 children.

The hospital administrator responsible for dealing with enquiries reported that a total of 231 enquiries were received and a total of 140 organs had been retained. It is debatable whether the figures were accurate as cataloguing all organs kept was time-consuming and might not have been complete. Parents also wanted additional information, for example as to 'whether the whole or part of the heart had ever been retained, what other tissue samples had been retained, why tissues had been retained, and when they were disposed of'.[4]

The Bristol Royal Infirmary was criticised for being inward-looking and reluctant to make changes which would benefit patients and families. The synopsis of the inquiry report states that:

'The story of the paediatric cardiac surgical service in Bristol is not an account of bad people. Nor is it an account of people who did not care, nor people who wilfully harmed patients. [But] it is an account of a hospital where there was a club culture; an imbalance of power, with too much control in the hands of a few individuals.'[5]

The report further states that:

'What was unusual about Bristol was that the systems and culture in place were such as to make open discussion and review more difficult. Staff were not encouraged to share their problems or to speak openly. Those who tried to raise concerns found it hard to have their voice heard.[5]

'Bristol had sufficient information from the 1980s onwards to challenge its own standards of care, had the surgeons and managers had the willingness to do so. Little, if any, of this information was available to the parents or to the public. Such information as was given to the parents was partial, confusing and unclear.'[5]

Many of the criticisms cited by the inquiry are equally relevant to such aspects as the management of post-mortem examinations and the removal and retention of human organs for clinical audit, teaching and research throughout the National Health Service (NHS). The inquiry report suggested that future 'patients in their journey through the healthcare system are entitled to be treated with respect and honesty and to be involved, wherever possible, in decisions about their care.'[5]

For the goal to be achieved, it would require effective communication between health professionals and patients and their relatives at all times. Doctors, nurses and managers must learn to communicate with each other effectively. There should be provision for stringent peer review where standards of treatment and care can be scrutinised. The NHS has been criticised by the Health Service Ombudsman in the past for its ineffective communication and the fact that the patient's voice is not heard.[6] In that regard it is worrying that nothing appears to have changed over the years and the public continues to struggle with health service bureaucracy and the problems of communicating with doctors and other health service personnel.

The 'club culture' referred to in the Bristol Inquiry report would prevent parents from speaking out about organ retention without consent as complaints would simply be overlooked by management. Parents complained about the way in which information concerning post-mortem examination was given. There was confusion among some who could not remember whether they were asked for consent. One mother said: 'I never gave permission for a post-mortem, I was simply told that one would happen.'[5] Another parent said: 'The hospital told us there would be a post-mortem as this was the usual practice, and we were sent the results. On the subject of organ retention, this was not addressed at the time.'[5]

The 'usual practice' might have arisen from a policy set out by the then South Western Regional Health Authority (SWRHA) in April 1991, which stated that 'all children who die in the perioperative period should have a post-mortem.'[4] This policy was an attempt to address the concerns about outcomes in paediatric cardiac surgery during the 1980s. However, the SWRHA categorically stated that 'retention of tissue for purposes other than to establish the cause of death is subject to the Human Tissue Act 1961. The constraints apply equally to clinical autopsies and those performed for the coroners.'[4]

Parents in Bristol from whom consent was sought (there was some debate over the substance of whether consent was in fact sought and obtained) also complained about the process by which it was sought. One of the parents said:

> 'I mean, we had literally come out of ITU and got back into this family room. I mean, a matter of minutes, five minutes at the outside, and there was this junior doctor suggesting that we should agree to a post-mortem. This had never been raised with us. ... If they had asked us [about a post-mortem] the night before our daughter's operation, and also after her death, I would have said – well, first of all, before the operation, I would have been affronted that they would have been seemingly dismissive, even before the operation, that she was going to die, so I would not have liked that. That is why I feel that well before the operation, when one is in a sober mind, it is far better approach that. But then after the operation, I would have found that difficult and I would have said no, but I do consider that well before we would have been in such a mind, in such a sensible mind, to have thought, yes, it would be a good thing, in the enforced event of death, for some good to be achieved.'[4]

The process of obtaining consent will be discussed in more detail in Chapter 10. The account presented here by the parent is not at all unusual. It might have been the first time the junior doctor had to ask a parent for post-mortem consent and perhaps he/she had never been taught how to do this important part of the 'house officer' job. It is seen by senior doctors as a job for the junior officer – learning the hard way. How can a junior doctor who has been qualified for a short time do one of the most difficult tasks effectively? The junior doctor may be embarrassed or he might disagree with the consent being asked for, but he is not in a position to argue with his senior. Perhaps he/she should have been accompanied by an experienced nurse, who could have helped to offer some sympathy and affection to the parent. As a result, the task of asking the parent to sign the consent form for post-mortem examination is often carried out too clinically, with no attempt by the doctor to stay with the parent once this has been done. The numbed and distressed parent is left alone either in a hospital corridor or a waiting room.

The Royal Liverpool Children's Inquiry

During the Bristol Inquiry, a professor of histopathology spoke of the benefits of retaining hearts for the purposes of study and teaching. Collections of hearts at various hospitals around the country had come to light in the interim report, which stated that: 'It was common practice, in Bristol and elsewhere, for human material removed during a post-mortem to be retained for long periods of time by pathologists. In a large number of cases, parents appear to have been unaware of this practice.'[4] The histopathologist estimated that the 'largest collection was at Alder Hey Children's Hospital, with approximately 2500 hearts.' He himself had built up a collection at the Royal Brompton Hospital of some 2000; there were collections at Great Ormond Street of 2000, at Birmingham Children's Hospital of about 1500, and other, smaller collections in Leeds, Bristol, Southampton, Newcastle and Manchester.[4] In the light of the disclosure of heart collections, members of the public started their own enquiries at their local hospitals. The responses from such enquiries pointed to the existence of substantial stores of human organs in Liverpool and in other locations throughout England and Wales.

In March 1999, the director of the Association of Community Health Councils for England and Wales wrote to the then Secretary of State for Health, Frank Dobson, pointing out that removal of organs and subsequent retention following post-mortem without consent and knowledge of relatives was unlawful and contrary to the provisions of the Human Tissue Act 1961.

In December 1999, Lord Hunt, the then Parliamentary Under-Secretary of State, set up an independent inquiry under the provision of Section 2 of the NHS Act 1977. The purpose was to investigate the removal, retention and disposal of human organs and tissues following post-mortem examination at Alder Hey Hospital (now known as the Liverpool Royal Children's NHS Trust).

The inquiry panel for Liverpool was appointed on 17 December 1999 and met five days later. It was chaired by Michael Redfern, QC. The central questions concerned the extent to which the Human Tissue Act 1961 had been complied with by the medical profession, and what had been the involvement of parents and family members in respect of the removal, retention and disposal of tissue (organs). The draft report was made available to the Department of Health in September 2000, which allowed the Chief Medical Officer to take appropriate action. The speed of this may indicate just how essential it was, in the face of public scandal, for there to be public examination of the practices in Liverpool.

When the final report was published on 30 January 2001, Alan Milburn, the then Secretary of State for Health, made the following statements to the House of Commons:

> The Redfern Report reveals a lack of respect and a failure to appreciate the circumstances which led to the taking of human material. For example, the Report cites entries about fetal material labelled with the words: 'Neck deeply lacerated. Pull it to pieces some time and reject.'

Some of these entries dated back many years. The number of organs retained by Alder Hey increased dramatically in the seven years following the appointment by the hospital and the University of Liverpool of Professor van Velzen in 1988, as Chair of Fetal and Infant Pathology…

During van Velzen's time at Alder Hey between 1988 and 1995, he systematically ordered the unethical and illegal stripping of every organ from every child who had had a post-mortem. He ignored parents' wishes even when they told him explicitly that they did not want a full post-mortem, let alone the retention of any of their child's organs.

According to the Report, van Velzen lied to parents. He lied to other doctors. He lied to hospital managers. He stole medical records. He falsified statistics and reports. And he encouraged other staff to do so.[7]

Milburn further said: 'At least 16 500 of these organs and tissues have been retained in apparent contravention of the law because they came about as a result of coroners' post-mortems, where organs should not have been kept beyond the time needed to establish cause of death.'[7]

The clinicians at Alder Hey 'did acknowledge in evidence the difficulties in reconciling their "paternalistic attitude" to the working of the then Human Tissue Act 1961. The doctors conceded that parents should have been asked about the retention of hearts. The failure to comply with the Act during the van Velzen years can be summarised by the question: would any parent not have objected if told that every organ of their child would be taken and in most cases left untouched for years without even an attempt at clinical histological examination?'[8]

The clinicians at Alder Hey were severely criticised by the Redfern Inquiry team for their failure to comply with the Human Tissue Act 1961. The Redfern Report concluded that 'there is abundant evidence of failure on the part of clinicians to make the requisite enquiries of parents to see if they objected. There is no evidence that the medical profession ever attempted to construe the Human Tissue Act.'[8] Even now we are told that these matters are not dealt with at any stage in the process of medical education and training.

Obviously, the inquiry could not possibly involve all those who have been affected by van Velzen's malpractice and what went on before his time. Many members of the public complained that there were organs and body parts which could not be traced due to the closure of hospitals during the last 20 to 30 years. As a result, many records have apparently been lost and therefore information has not been available to answer the public's enquiries. However, information should be available for those who died more recently, say within the last five to 10 years. A very distressed mother and father at one of the public meetings enquired about the whereabouts of the whole body of one of their twins, who died soon after birth. It was claimed by the parents that one of the twins was sent away to another country for research.[9] A further incident of a similar nature was brought to the attention of the Retained Organs Commission. A very distressed woman said she had been told 17 years ago that her twins had been buried, only to discover that only one had been laid to rest and there was no trace of the other.[9] Of course, if post-mortems had not so often involved lack of transparency, these consequent problems would not have arisen.

Many parents lost their child during pregnancy and their queries concerning whether the remains had been kept by the hospital were confirmed by the inquiry team. The Redfern team found a fetal collection at the Institute of Child Health. 'The fetal collection at the ICH was recorded in February 2000 as containing 1564 stillbirths or pre-viable fetuses including 52 late premature or term fetuses, although none since 1973. The store of primarily intact fetal tissue started in 1955 with identification detail from 1975 and ceased in 1992. The collection was started by Dr Hay. At one stage the collection contained a total of 3575 fetuses but in the three years before transferring to the new Institute of Child Health building a substantial number were incinerated.'[8]

Following Professor van Velzen's arrival in 1988, 'a significant amount of fetal material, largely deriving from miscarriage and therapeutic termination, was sent to his unit for histology and subsequent sensitive disposal. This was essentially a regional service for fetal abnormalities and approximately 100 fetuses per year would be received.'[8] (It is important to note here that fetuses from other hospitals of the same region would be sent to van Velzen's unit). 'Due to Professor van Velzen's failure to attend to the fetal pathology service, a backlog built up and was never resolved. In December 1999, 445 fetuses were retained at Myrtle Street dating back to 1989–91. Of the 445 fetuses, 198 were intact. In February 2000, a further 30 fetuses were identified.'[8]

In addition to the fetal collection, 22 body parts from 15 children, 13 heads/parts of heads from children from a few days old to 11 years of age dating back to the 1960s, and 22 heads from late premature/term fetuses were also found. There were two containers with a whole body of a child in one and the separated head in the other. 'Perhaps the most disturbing specimen is that of the head of a boy aged 11 years. The most recent specimen was obtained in 1973.'[10]

The Redfern Inquiry did find during its investigation documentary evidence of transferring body parts from one part of the UK to another: a number of hospitals supplied body parts, once consent had been provided for research purposes. It is not clear whether the reference made to consent was in fact written consent from the parents concerned or from the transferring authorities.[8]

Was it possible that whole bodies could have been sent to other parts of the UK and to other countries outside the UK for research purposes? For example, it was reported during the Redfern Inquiry that on 18 September 2000 the Canadian police had:

'…seized 13 boxes of what appeared to be internal organs. They had been contacted by staff at a storage company who were removing items stored by Professor van Velzen on leaving Canada in 1998. The contracted period for storage in the warehouse had expired and the large wooden crate, which contained the boxes, had been turned over to auction. Testing of the organs revealed that in 12 of the boxes there were animal organs and in the last box human organs. The Canadian police believe that they relate to two young children but do not link them to children in the United Kingdom. Professor van Velzen's legal representatives also have indicated that the organs do not originate from the United Kingdom. However, a number of original medical records relating to children at Alder Hey were discovered, some dating back to the 1970s.'[10]

Some family members believed that their children's eyes had been removed as their sockets were sunken when the bodies were seen in the mortuary or in the chapel of rest. At the CMO Summit one of the parents said: 'When we [the parent and friend] opened the cupboard there were three jars: one with babies' hearts, one with babies' lungs, and one looked like peas. When I looked closely, they were eyes.'[3]

The CMO Summit was called by the Chief Medical Officer against the background of the anger and concerns expressed by parents and families in Bristol and Liverpool. The Summit was held on 11 January 2001 at the Queen Elizabeth II Conference Centre in London. Oral presentations were given by parents and relatives, voluntary organisations such as PITY II (Parents who have Interred their Young Twice), NACOR (The National Committee Relating to Organs Retention), the Bristol Heart Children Action Group, the Child Bereavement Trust, scientific, research and professional bodies, representatives of the Registrar of the London Beth Din and the Muslim Council of Britain and the Muslim Doctors and Dentists Association, Hospital Chaplaincies Council, the Patient Liaison Group of the Royal College of Pathologists. Written evidence from the above was also submitted to the Summit.

It would appear that the evidence presented by the families above to the CMO Summit could be confirmed as there was a formal research grant application submitted on 8 March 1994 to the Wellcome Trust by Professor Grierson, Professor van Velzen and Dr Howard. The application stated that: 'A total of 150 fetal and infant eyes are available to us at present and have been introduced into the database as part of our pilot feasibility investigation. The specimens range from the second fetal month to term and then there are eyes from neonates and infants up to four years of age... Between one and two suitable specimens come to the Department of Fetal and Infant Pathology each week so that it is our expectation to have an additional 50–100 specimens per year for the optic nerve investigations.'[10]

The Dean of the Medical School, Professor Johnson, was unaware of the fetal collection until he was told by the head of Department of Medicine on 7 December 1999. Professor Johnson subsequently ordered an inventory of the collection to be carried out and the report was submitted to the Alder Hey Inquiry on 24 March 2000. The collection had begun with a pilot study by Professor Ian Grierson and Dr Howard in 1993 which had resulted in a successful application for a Wellcome Trust grant. He was assured that the eyeballs were taken from fetuses, and not from neonates or older children. However, documents obtained by the inquiry team could not rule out the possibility that eyes had in fact been taken from children at post-mortem examinations and there was 'no evidence of any consent, other than the usual consent obtained at the time of post-mortem'.[10] Evidence from the report would support the parents' view that eyes from children were deliberately taken without permission. Some of the eyes were used for study. The surplus was left in jars.

Even if one wants to be benevolent towards individual doctors and the medical profession, there is no intelligent explanation to offer for using eyes in this way and leaving them in jars. The problem is that even now some doctors will still insist that there was no wrongdoing. Collecting human organs for the sake of collecting may just be a medical custom similar to those of other collectors. The habit of collecting for the 'just in case' situation can be referred to as a collector phenomenon without a rational base. The collector phenomenon could be described as an insatiable desire to possess objects of perceived value, but the objects may or may not have value at present or in the future. It could also be described as an obsession. The term can best be exemplified by a discussion between a group of senior doctors and the author a few years ago when the issue of brain research was raised. The group of academic clinicians was asked whether there was a limit to the number of brains that would be needed for the project. The response was: 'We could always use normal brains as controls.' However, the Royal Liverpool Children's Inquiry shows that many human remains were never used for the said purpose of research.

One cannot imagine what the feelings of these collectors of children's body parts and heads would be if the specimens were from their own children. One might try to resist a feeling of revulsion at the collecting practice, but one cannot. It is difficult to understand the rationality of those who were involved in the collections. One can only assume the body parts were collected in the interests of science and teaching. From the parents' point of view, the disclosure made by the Alder Hey Inquiry demonstrates the unsatisfactory and inhumane nature of pathology practice in Liverpool and throughout the rest of the UK. One can see why the public in Liverpool demanded a change in the law.

Organ retention in adults

The Isaacs Inquiry and Report

It had become clear that the practice of removing and retaining organs following post-mortem examination without the consent and knowledge of parents and families was widespread,[3,4,5,8,10,11] and that it also applied to dead adults. At public meetings of the Retained Organs Commission, families often expressed their anger at this practice.

The Isaacs Inquiry,[12] although concerned primarily with one deceased male adult whose brain was removed and retained during post-mortem without the knowledge and consent of the family, led to the disclosure of many adult cases of brains being removed for research and clinical purposes.

The inquiry was instigated by Mrs Elaine Isaacs following her discovery in April 2000 that her late husband's brain had been removed without her knowledge and consent during a post-mortem that took place in February 1987, and had been sent to Manchester University for research. The report states that 'had Mr Isaacs' family been aware at that time of the retention of any of Mr Isaacs' organs, this would have been vigorously opposed.'[12]

Mrs Isaacs submitted a detailed account at the CMO Summit on 11 January 2001. Following debate in the House of Commons on 30 January 2001, Mrs Isaacs' son wrote to the then Secretary of State for Health, Alan Milburn, requesting an investigation into what had occurred following the death of his father.

On 29 July 2001, Her Majesty's Inspector of Anatomy was appointed by the Secretary of State to investigate Mr Isaacs' death and in particular the retention and intended use for research of his brain. The terms of reference were: to investigate and document the procedures and circumstances which led to the removal and retention of organs of the late Cyril Mark Isaacs during the autopsy performed at Prestwich Mortuary on 27 February 1987; to investigate what subsequently happened to the organ removed and retained; to review whether similar removals of organs occurred at other public mortuaries after deaths outside hospitals; to examine these events in the light of clinical and ethical policies, relevant legislation, religious beliefs, and the expectation and rights of relatives; to report conclusions and recommendations to the Secretary of State for Health.[12]

The Isaacs Inquiry covered the period 1985 to 1995. Its report found that 'in 1985 the public was largely unaware of what happened during a post-mortem and of the possibility of organ and tissue retention. Pathologists, morticians and others were aware of the details but rarely discussed these with relatives.'[12] The Isaacs Report also covered other aspects of post-mortem and pathology practices and matters relating to research and therapeutic programmes such as: research on brains retained at post-mortem; the research programme at the departments of physiology and psychiatry at Manchester University (the 'joint programme'); research at other locations on brains from coroners' cases; the collection and use of brains for teaching; brain retention and the special hospitals (e.g. Ashworth Hospital, Broadmoor Hospital, etc where offenders for serious crimes are held in custody. All deaths in the special hospitals and where deaths are automatically reported to the coroner, whether or not there are any suspicious circumstances); the involvement of research-funding organisations and Royal Colleges; attitudes to post-mortems and organ retention; the importance of post-mortem research to the future of healthcare and consequent changes and the need for further change.

Under the heading 'Research on brains at post-mortem', the Isaacs Report considered the national pituitary collection programme, which began as a Medical Research Council-funded research project before the enactment of the Human Tissue Act in 1961. The legality of retaining tissues on the authority of the coroner was questioned by a member of the MRC Human Pituitary Collection Committee at a meeting held in December 1977. He said that 'he had been approached by a number of pathologists supplying pituitaries who were disturbed by the differences in procedure between hospital post-mortems and coroners' post-mortems regarding the permission of relatives for the removal of tissues. Some pathologists were uneasy about the situation and were concerned about possible adverse publicity.'[12] However, after discussion the committee agreed that the spirit of the Human Tissue Act 1961 was not being broken as the 'coroners were in legal possession of the bodies of those whose deaths were reported to them, they were legally entitled to say whether human tissues (i.e. pituitaries) could be taken from the bodies and used for medical education and research...DHSS would discuss and clarify with the Home Office the whole situation.'[12] The practice of collecting human pituitaries from dead persons was guided by the Health Circular (HC77)28[13], which was issued to the NHS in August 1977, stating that 'specific consent is not required by the Act' (the Human Tissue Act 1961) for the removal of pituitaries for the national collection programme.

The law governing post-mortem examinations, and the interpretation and application of the Human Tissue Act 1961 for teaching and research, were two fundamental areas which emerged as needing scrutiny as a result of the investigation of one case, that of Mr Isaacs. The University of Manchester and the

Prestwich Mortuary were part of that investigation. The Isaacs Report also examined thoroughly other locations involved in brain research from coroners' cases, such as the Cambridge Brain Bank, Queen's Medical Centre in Nottingham and Radcliffe Infirmary in Oxford, and the practice of brain retention from post-mortems after death in special hospitals such as Ashworth, Broadmoor and Rampton. During the course of the Isaacs Inquiry, members of the public often raised their concern with the Retained Organs Commission about the legality of brain retention.

Other aspects such as research funding organisations, Royal Colleges and research governance, including Local Research Ethics Committees (LRECs), were examined by HM Inspector of Anatomy. The role of government departments, in particular the Department of Health, the medical profession, the research community including the MRC, individual medical practitioners and researchers, the funding organisations, and those who approve and monitor research were also considered in the Isaacs Report.

The medical and research communities appear, according to the Isaacs Inquiry, to have failed to merit public trust. For example, the investigation carried out at the Queen's Medical Centre, Nottingham revealed that 'approximately 1700 brains from coroners' cases are retained in the collection. ...These have been accumulated mostly since 1970 but the oldest brain was retained in 1967. All the brains were obtained or referred from other hospitals for diagnosis. None was collected solely for research.'[12]

The Isaacs Report further stated that 'the relatives, with a few exceptions, had no way of knowing that the brains had been retained after a coroner's post-mortem. The relatives were not informed when brains were disposed of.'[12] There are other examples in the report which suggest that families have also been either intentionally or unintentionally deceived about the nature of post-mortem examination and the use of brains for research or other purposes. To what extent paternalism can be used as a defence is difficult to judge. Deceit is surely unethical.

The Isaacs case and others show that respect for religious beliefs and families' wishes were grossly ignored. Without the resolve of the Isaacs family, the truth about the practice and attitudes involved in brain collections would not have been so fully revealed. From the inquiries and reports discussed in this book there is some revelation of how many families' humanity was bypassed by the system. If the practice were to be left unreformed, how many more families would suffer?

Issues of research governance and accountability

The Isaacs Inquiry and Report directed a spotlight on research governance and the lack of rigorous monitoring mechanisms while the research is in progress. It has been the personal observation of the author that the standards of approval mechanisms vary in practice. I have been troubled in the past by my research students' concerns, following their attendance at LREC meetings, about the process by which approval is given to research proposals, as they often expressed their anxiety regarding the competence with which their proposals were scrutinised by LREC members. (I would hasten to add that the majority of my research students received approval at their first attempt and the remaining applications needed some minor amendments.) Members of LRECs from various locations in the UK often missed vital information that was explained in the proposals and therefore irrelevant questions were asked. The students had the distinct impression that their paperwork had not been read by some members before their meeting. For example, some members would ask 'Have you discussed your sample size with the statistician?' in spite of the fact that it was clearly spelled out in a section of the application form.

I share my students' anxiety about the approval process and should like to give an example here to illustrate my own concerns. About three years ago, I attended a research and ethics committee meeting to consider 20 proposals submitted by nurses, doctors and academics. (Some of the proposals submitted for approval had been approved by another committee, of which the person referred to below was a member.) One of the committee members (who happened to be a GP) arrived late without his papers. Apparently he had not read the proposals as he had just come back from holiday. His papers were still in his office. What was the purpose of his attendance? Coincidentally, some of the proposals put to our committee for consideration, which as mentioned above had previously been approved by another LREC (as the applicants needed approval from more than one committee), were rejected.

Since then, I have often wondered how effective is the approval process. Are all proposals studied by the members of the committees prior to approval meetings? Are proposals passed on the nod by busy members if the proposer is respected? (That was the case when I attended some European Union grant application meetings.) A more stringent procedure for the appointment of appropriately qualified members may need to be imposed centrally, and members may need to be subject to annual review by external assessors. Lay member appointments to committees should overcome possible 'club culture' as implied in the Bristol Royal Infirmary Inquiry. Indeed, reform is now under way. Of course, more central controls are not exactly sought by doctors today, yet systems need to improve at the critical points. Nor is it the case that doctors and researchers need to be censured, but rather that they need recognition, and even perhaps some compensation, for ethics committee work and the use of their time to study proposals.

The moral responsibility of the research ethics committees, government departments, high-profile research institutions and researchers cannot be overlooked. Funders of research such as the MRC and charities should play a key role in keeping the research institutions and individual researchers mindful of these aspects.

The Bristol, Alder Hey and Isaacs Inquiries confirmed the supposition that clinicians had failed to comply with the Act of Parliament dealing with the use of the deceased body for medical purposes. Good law should provide a good synthesis of intention and regulation; this may have been imperfect in the 1961 Act. Doctors had apparently ignored the intention and the letter of the law although, crucially, quite what any legal implications this might have, for aggrieved families in particular, was, and is, unclear and beyond the scope of this book. In addition, solicited and unsolicited sources, such as those published in the press and oral evidence presented by families at public meetings of the Retained Organs Commission, echoed the findings of the inquiries.

The Retained Organs Commission was established by the Secretary of State for Health on 1 April 2001 as a special health authority following the publication of the Redfern Report and on the recommendation of the Chief Medical Officer. The key tasks of the Commission were to work in partnership with families, the public and professionals on issues relating to organ retention; to oversee the proper return of retained organs and tissue to families who request it; to consult on and propose a regulatory framework for museum and archives of human tissue, and to advise government ministers about the changes needed in the law relating to organ retention and post-mortem examinations.[14] The fear of families that organs and body parts had been removed without their knowledge and permission was founded. The Chief Medical Officer further confirmed that, in his process of inquiry, the practice of removing organs and body parts was not unique to the three hospitals; it was widespread throughout hospitals in England and had gone on for many years.

The issue of laws lacking in clarity emerged constantly between 2001 and 2004 during the life of the Retained Organs Commission. Laws which are flawed tend to be open to subjective interpretation by individual practitioners and researchers who, while not being in any sense intentionally bad, and having among their priorities scientific progress, may lack a certain desirable interest in social and ethical aspects. It emerged in one of these inquiries that government departments interpreted the law for the benefit of the research community, under the guise of 'public interest or public good'. The public was right in that the laws regulating this aspect of medical practice did not serve to protect the vulnerable. Part of future legislation should address the issue of punishment for those misguided doctors who wilfully intend to pursue their own objectives without attention to ethics or regulations. Now that, unfortunately, there have been disconcerting cases that undermine trust in the medical profession – from Bristol to Alder Hey and on to problems of expert medical witnesses and still further to Shipman – the testimony of families and relatives who suffered should be taken into serious consideration in decisions regarding the nature of ethical standards and the legal framework.

Author's reflection

During the last three years I have often been troubled by some of the phrases used by some doctors, hospital chaplains and those associated with the health service. The commonest remarks amount to: 'What do we [doctors] have to apologise for? Why do we [the health service] spend so much money on the dead? Money could be better spent on research and in the treatment of cancer patients.' Nurses and those staffing the organ retention helpline have been more sympathetic and in tune with the feelings of those who have suffered hurt and grief, or at least they have shown awareness of others.

The Alder Hey experience sparked off a range of reactions and responses. The way that people's lives were touched was both quite simple, since it brought a revival of grief and a deep sense of being wrongly treated, and more complex, because some attitudes towards death and the human body appeared to be at variance with an almost post-religious society that is seen as increasingly materialistic. The keen need to rebury the dead in as complete a state as possible, perhaps more than once, with newly restored parts that had been retained, is an example of this. Clearly there are human ethical issues at work. It is the victims' families alone who offer any prospect of understanding these issues – if we are interested in listening to and respecting what they have to say. After all, we have a limited capacity to understand their pain because we probably have little to compare it with, let alone the capacity to empathise completely.

So far, one does not get the impression that lessons have been learned. The past is a good teacher as it offers opportunities for reflection. It can help us find ways of managing our lives or affairs more effectively. The question is, does the health service want people to speak openly about the service delivered? How often are patients and relatives asked about their experiences as users? Even if there were opportunities for patients and relatives to exchange views, would the suggestions be implemented? There do not appear to have been any effective feedback mechanisms for patients and relatives to communicate their views about the health service and the way health professionals behave. If there had been, then concerns such as those raised by the families in Bristol, Liverpool and elsewhere might have been met far earlier. The health service has always functioned as predominantly a one-way service: deliver care without necessarily seeking feedback from patients. As a result, issues about standards of care are not brought out into the open.

At a public meeting held in Liverpool, some parents were talking about their recent experiences. Others referred to incidents which happened 20 years or so ago and some gave their personal account of events as far back as 50 years ago. From the observer's point of view, all the personal accounts of organ retention at Alder Hey seemed as recent as yesterday and the emotions were visibly raw. Some of those who did not want to speak or could not bring themselves to talk about their experiences publicly chose to write. One parent kept a history of a child who had died 27 years ago: 'Yes, time has healed my grief, the emptiness and the feelings of failure and bitterness, but I will never forget Philip, or the fact that for thirty-six hours, I was his mother and we were a family.' This mother further said: 'Never in my darkest and saddest times over twenty-seven years did I for one moment think, or even imagine, that any of Philip's organs were kept at the hospital [Addenbrooke's Hospital, Cambridge]. I had always believed that he had been cremated and laid to rest...'[15]

The emotions felt by these parents were by no means unique to Liverpool. Parents' worlds were turned upside down by those very people whom they had looked up to in the past. They now believed the world of medicine to be a cruel place.

Of course it is not just the case that there has been confrontation between 'them and us', with the families on one side and medical and legal professionals on the other. There are also clear differences of attitude, and apparently of values, between the families who were victims at Alder Hey and elsewhere, and much of the rest of the population.

Religious differences, while they may explain some individual points of view, do not explain the division. Those who have not had the experience of being victims of the system cannot understand the extent of the problem. They may go on to advocate the unrestricted medical use of organs and other tissue from the bodies of individuals unless the dead person has specifically opted out. At some future time this may turn out to be – once there is more understanding and regard for the paramount need to make the procedures work well – what

is required by the majority of people in a democracy, and be broadly acceptable to society. What we appear to have now is a degree of polarity of views
based on experience. At present, the victims' experience is beyond the understanding of some doctors and members of other health professions.

I spoke briefly about empathy in Chapter 1, but it is difficult to empathise if
one cannot enter into the realm of the other person's world. One is more able
to understand the feelings of losing a close friend or a relative if one has had
experience of bereavement. I surveyed the attitudes of Church of England ministers and Catholic priests towards a woman subject a few years ago. The Catholic
priests who responded to my survey showed little or no understanding at all and
some disregarded the subject almost out of hand. Some among the Church of
England clerics who took part in the study, especially those who were married
and had been through the same experience, were a great deal more sympathetic.
In a similar way, doctors and others indirectly connected with the organ retention scandal may show no remorse or sympathy towards the Liverpool families.

Educational awareness campaigns may achieve some desired effects, but in
the first place the mindset of these individuals needs to be changed. I do not
believe legislation alone can influence the mindset either. It might even encourage doctors and healthcare managers to be more intransigent. The public is the
real change agent in healthcare matters as they can and must speak up and
speak out about their experiences and grievances. To achieve change in the NHS
through public pressure, the public must be knowledgeable in health matters
and prepared to raise objections to treatment prescribed and the manner in
which complaints are dealt with. Surely this is an area where money should be
spent to empower the public to be effective change agents?

There appears to be a high level of agreement among families who have direct
experience of organ retention. Among the medical profession, however,
opinions are varied and again are polarised. Some responses from other professional groups involved in welfare and social care, including the religious, have
been surprising. Some Church of England ministers, Roman Catholic priests and
hospital chaplains appear to believe that the 'paternalism' of doctors' actions is
altogether to the benefit of patients. During a conversation at a hospital trust
meeting, one hospital chaplain gave his view:

> 'Medical paternalism was acceptable 30 to 40 years ago because the public
> had faith in the doctors. I don't see anything wrong in that. After all, the
> doctors know what is best for the patients. We have entered into a new
> era now where the public knows more about medical science and expects
> more from the doctors and questions everything.'
>
> (Author's personal notes, 2002)

It is understandable that a minister of religion should sympathise with the
procedures of the genuinely caring medical profession. Most ministers of religion
work in the tradition of living faiths that adapt their religious philosophy to fit,
albeit slowly, the changing world. A culture of paternalism in the NHS may
extend further than the medical profession itself. It may be shared by managers
and administrators, the media and some members of the public, and perhaps
by some ethicists.

There was such an atmosphere of secrecy, and a consequent impression of
deceit, in the aftermath of the organ retention and post-mortem disclosures that

confrontation between the doctors and families was inevitable. The families were bound to become 'the accusers' and the doctors 'the accused'. Reconciliation is only achievable if common ground is identified. The aims of the NHS to provide the best possible treatment would of course be part of this. There might also be a reassessment of ethics so that ideas of what is acceptable – and indeed what is objectionable – are agreed. This could have less to do with strictly rational notions of scientific progress, and more to do with understanding that a breakdown in trust owing to deception in practice, however well-meaning, demands more emphasis on observing decency and according respect.

Of course, post-mortem examinations would contribute to a better understanding of diseases and treatments if they were to be carried out according to strict rules and required standards. As we have seen, many within the medical profession, especially surgeons and pathologists, considered that the collection and retention of human specimens without prior consent and discussion was quite simply carried out in the best interests of the patients and their families – a proper part of benign medical paternalism, intended to protect the relatives from the further upset and distress that would be involved in asking for consent and divulging distressing details. After the Bristol Inquiry disclosure that there were collections of organs in the health service, some doctors expressed surprise that the public was angry and that there were demands for action from the government.

Those with a medico-scientific viewpoint could not understand why what had long been standard practice was suddenly regarded as so offensive. From their perspective, the body is a machine for living and over the last 300 years the scientific study of dead bodies has been pursued in order to help future living patients. Death has offered a unique opportunity to study the anatomy and physiology of both the normal and diseased human body[16] and these endeavours were clearly undertaken in the interests of science and in the interests of the public.

Some medical practitioners would not see the practice adopted in the past as problematic, since they do not believe present standards of practice should be used to judge past action. In their view, no one would doubt the importance of proper informed consent. However, standards change over time. The form of consent that was entirely acceptable 30 years ago might cause outrage today, but that does not necessarily mean that it was inappropriate then. It is quite wrong to judge, in retrospective analysis, the actions of 10, 20 or 30 years ago by today's standards.[17]

There are also those among the medical profession who expressed regret and offered sympathy. They recognised that the practice in the past was undesirable and caused unnecessary grief to the bereaved families. For example, the Forensic Society and the British Neuropathology Society submitted the following written responses to the CMO Summit:

> The medical profession in the United Kingdom has recently suffered from a spate of highly publicised incidents that have shaken public confidence. In particular, the scandal over the retention of children's body parts collected at post-mortem examination at Bristol Royal Infirmary and in children's hospitals in Birmingham, Liverpool and Glasgow had a major adverse effect on the public perception of the medical profession.[18]

The latest discovery of brains retained without their relatives' knowledge and agreement has caused further distress.

To restore public confidence, a more sensitive, patient-centred mechanism for obtaining agreement to organ retention is indicated.[19]

Some views reflect the suggestion that doctors were victims of poorly written and badly applied law. Such an assertion could contribute to discussions of the reform of existing laws governing post-mortem examinations and the use of body parts for education and research. Further, the Adler Hey scandal was seen by some doctors as providing 'a convenient stick with which to beat the medical profession...and this cynical manipulation of morbid anxieties is distressing to the bereaved, demoralising to hospital staff and damaging to medicine.'[15] The doctors were hurt, but do they share pain comparable to that suffered by the families?

The reflections of the families are very different. They see their rights as having been violated; that they have been badly treated by the medical profession and let down by the National Health Service; that they have been lied to and their lives intruded upon. From the families' point of view, their children and relatives have been badly treated after death. The medical profession and the health service have failed to observe the principle of human respect towards both the living and the dead. For example, the disposal of human body parts after post-mortem examination, by means of incineration of clinical waste, is considered by families to be totally inappropriate and disrespectful. Families are hurt by their experience and feel they are not understood. If there is any possible deficit in their logic, their feelings about ethical issues are formed by the impeccable authority of experience.

A couple appearing on television in 2004 made a profound statement after losing their mother in a coach crash, which could illustrate the feelings of an Alder Hey or other family. One of them said:

'I don't think he [the coach driver] knows what we've been through. He wouldn't understand the hurt and pain we've lived through and are living through. Our grief and experience will stay with us for the rest of our lives.'

(Author's personal notes, 2004)

The statement above is obvious, but this does not mean that nothing can be learned from it. People without the same experience cannot possibly understand the sufferers' feelings about their loss. By appearing on television the couple were caught up in another chapter of the publicised tragedy of a newsworthy road accident. For them, the loss of their mother was compounded by the circumstances. The retained-organ families of Liverpool, Bristol, Birmingham, Glasgow and other parts of the UK, like that bereaved couple, were caught up in doubled pain. There was the death (often of a child) and also the scandal of concealed organ retention which, once it was exposed, went under a spotlight of public and legal attention. Possibly in both cases there are people who would blame the sufferers themselves for the media interest. That again is an indication that it may be easier to criticise than to empathise. A written statement submitted to the CMO Summit by a parent said:

'...I know it is an overused term to say that words cannot express the pain of losing a child, or just how it feels to discover that someone has decided that they have more right to take parts of your child without asking or even gaining permission, but I do and can express it into adequate words if only people would listen. People have said to me that the medical profession see things differently, as if that justifies it or excuses them, but I think that is frightening in itself. I also wonder how the people who tell me this or the doctors themselves would feel if it was their child.'[20]

Upon reading this quote it is easy to understand that families are aggrieved that no one in the health service appeared to understand them, so that consequently their concerns were not heard. Can tragic experience be shared with others? Sharing experience or achieving empathy requires mutual understanding of a high order; but given the traditional practices in the health service, that is a lot to ask. In principle, of course, empathy is possible even if the starting point of each individual is different – provided there is a will to change. The health professional is often criticised by patients for failing to see things from their point of view. Admittedly, maybe health professionals require a certain degree of emotional detachment in order to function effectively. To empathise, one needs to step into the other person's shoes, which is precisely the challenge issued by parents who submitted their testimonies to the CMO Summit. Indeed, they eloquently answered the question, 'Why all the fuss?'

References

1   Professor John Hay's obituary. *The Times*, 20 January 2004: 41.
2   Department of Health. Human bodies, Human Choices: the law on human organs and tissue in England and Wales. A consultation report. London: Department of Health Publications; 2002.
3   Department of Health. Chief Medical Officer's Summit: evidence documentation. The Queen Elizabeth Conference Centre. 11 January 2001. London: Department of Health; 2001; Ref: OR-222.
4   The Bristol Royal Infirmary Inquiry. The Report of the Inquiry into the Management of Care of Children Receiving Complex Heart Surgery at the Bristol Royal Infirmary: interim report. London: Central Office of Information; 2000.
5   The Bristol Royal Infirmary Inquiry. The Report of the Public Inquiry into Children's Heart Surgery at the Bristol Royal Infirmary, 1984–1995. Learning from Bristol. London: The Stationery Office; 2001. © Crown copyright.
6   The National Health Service Commissioner's Report – Annual reports 1977–1985. London: HMSO. © Crown copyright.
7   House of Commons. Royal Liverpool Children's Inquiry Report published today. Statement to the House of Commons by Health Secretary Alan Milburn. House of Commons, 30 January 2001.
8   The Royal Liverpool Children's Inquiry. The Royal Liverpool Children's Inquiry Report: summary and recommendations. London: The Stationery Office Ltd; 2001.
9   The NHS Retained Organs Commission. Minutes of the 3rd meeting. Liverpool; London: The NHS Organs Retention Commission; 2001.
10   The Royal Liverpool Children's Inquiry. The Royal Liverpool Children's Inquiry Report. London: The Stationery Office; 2001.

11 Department of Health. Report of a Census of Organs and Tissues Retained by the Pathology Service Conducted in 2000 by the Chief Medical Officer. London: The Stationery Office Ltd; 2001.

12 The Isaacs Inquiry. The Isaacs Report: the investigation of events that followed the death of Cyril Mark Isaacs. London: The Stationery Office Ltd; 2003.

13 Department of Health and Social Security (DHSS) HC(77)28. Removal of human tissue at post mortem examination – Human Tissue Act 1961. London: DHSS; 1977.

14 The Retained Organs Commission. Annual Report 2002–2003. London: The Retained Organs Commission; 2003.

15 Freeman AD. My grief for Philip. A case submitted by a member of the public to the NHS Retained Organs Commission in February 2003. London: The NHS Retained Organs Commission; 2003.

16 Fitzpatrick M. Second opinion [accessed Oct 2002]. Available from: file//A:\spiked-health%/20%20column%20%20second%20opinion.htm.

17 Department of Health. Chief Medical Officer's Summit: evidence documentation. London: Department of Health; 2001; 223 -OR.

18 Ibid. 2001. Written evidence submitted by the British Neuropathology Society. Sheffield: 219 -OR.

19 Ibid. 2001Written evidence submitted by the Forensic Science Society. Harrogate: 219 -OR.

20 Ibid. 2001; Evidence submitted by a parent. 225 -OR.

Chapter 6

Misinterpreting the rules of post-mortem examination and the Human Tissue Act 1961

Public perceptions of post-mortem examination

The medical profession strongly supports the principle that post-mortem examinations are intended to ascertain the cause of death. Despite this, many relatives have had to search for this evidence, which should have been given by doctors at the end of the examination process. An anonymous speaker at one of the Retained Organs Commission meetings, whose father died when she was 11 years old, said: 'I have spent my entire life in lengthy and inconclusive research into the causes and circumstance of my father's death.'[1] This involved a hereditary condition and so the evidence gathered could have been especially important for future generations.

A parent in Liverpool, who again wished to be unnamed, said: 'In many instances in Liverpool, post-mortems have not been written up, and in many cases genetic advice [which is often argued by doctors and pathologists to be one of the important reasons for post-mortems] has not been given to at-risk parents.'[2]

One can immediately discern that the medical profession and the public are at variance over the purpose and benefit of post-mortem examination. It was often argued most strongly by pathologists and doctors at public meetings during 2001–2004 that findings obtained from post-mortem examinations would allow them to study and understand inherited conditions, so that individuals concerned could then be advised in order to make informed decisions. A member of the public belonging to a family support group said that she had never come across anyone who had benefited from genetic advice obtained at post-mortem. In her personal experience she had not been advised of further risk. This was backed up by another person present who said: 'There has been a lack of feedback to families, who have gone on to have further children who have suffered from the same disease.'[3]

For some, the quest for explanations and basic information has been going on for 40 to 50 years, and for others the search has just started. A discussion took place between the author and a woman whose husband had died about 35 years earlier. She said no one had explained the meaning of congestive heart failure and pulmonary oedema, reported in her husband's death certificate. This is an example of how professionals have in the past failed to grasp that people often want to be given full information, but may need help in understanding it. It does not suffice to say they cannot grasp what a particular condition entails and so should not be burdened with explanation. The woman went on to say in respect of the post-mortem: 'Since my husband died from heart failure, why was an autopsy required when the cause was known? I can understand why the doctors wanted to look at the heart, but why did they want to look at his brain and other organs?' She saw no legitimate reason for this, let alone why they were retained. More importantly, she had not been consulted. Neither was she informed of the results of the examination. For her, further time has been spent trying to find out from the health service where her husband's heart, brain and other organs were kept after his post-mortem. Her experience, which is not rare, contributed to an unfortunate impression that doctors and health service managers had been actively dishonest.

Since there is often some confusion about the differences between hospital-based and coroners' post-mortem examinations, it would be educative to describe what a post-mortem examination entails, the two types of examination, the law that governs this particular practice, and the rights of the public in these circumstances.

Distinctions between hospital-based and coroners' post-mortem examinations

After a person has died, whether in hospital or at home, a medical practitioner is required to examine the deceased and certify the cause of death. If the doctor is satisfied with the cause of death, then a death certificate is signed, allowing the family to register the death with the Registrar of Births and Deaths. Funeral arrangements can then be made.

In most cases the cause of death is clear-cut. Where it is not clear-cut or cannot be easily explained, or the circumstances in which the person is found dead are suspicious, the doctor is obliged by law to refer the death to the coroner. The authority of the coroner is governed by the Coroners Rules 1984 and the Coroners Act 1988. The Coroners Rules derive their authority from the Coroners Act.

'The majority of deaths referred to coroners are sudden and unexpected deaths of unknown cause.'[4] In a small number of cases, 'the cause will be known when deaths are reported, e.g. road traffic accidents, [but] the coroner still needs to satisfy the Coroners Rule 36 to identify how the deceased came by his death. Rule 36 of the Coroners Act 1988 requires the coroner to identify (a) who the deceased was, (b) how, when and where the deceased came by her or his death, and (c) the particulars for the time being required by the Registration Acts to be registered concerning the death.'[4]

All deaths which happen in police or prison custody or in special hospitals, e.g. Rampton, are referred to the coroner. Referrals to the coroner may also be made by families where the relatives suspect that the cause of death is directly related to the treatment given. Once deaths are referred for investigation, the deceased's relatives have no legal right to challenge any decisions made by the coroner. However, the relatives should be informed by the coroner of where and when the investigation will take place and who will carry out the post-mortem examination, if required.

For deaths of unknown cause, the coroner will need to determine whether the cause of death can be 'satisfactorily established by reference to the deceased's existing medical condition(s).'[4] If the deceased's medical history provides sufficient information to satisfy the coroner, then a post-mortem should not be necessary. However, the coroner's right to insist on a post-mortem is essentially to safeguard the public. If a post-mortem is required, the coroner will appoint a qualified medical practitioner to carry out the examination.

In other cases of sudden and unexpected death, an inquest may be ordered by the coroner without having recourse to a post-mortem examination, provided that the information obtained from such an inquiry reveals the cause of death satisfactorily. However, not every sudden and unexpected death requires an inquest. The position paper *Reforming the Coroner and Death Certification Service*, published by the Home Office in 2004, states that: 'If the death was sudden and unexpected, but the coroner is satisfied as a result of his or her inquiries that the death was due to natural causes, no inquest is required.'[5] Where death appears to have been violent or unnatural an inquest must be held. If an inquest is held, the coroner, and the jury in certain cases, is responsible for ascertaining who has died, when and how.

The coroner's inquest may be held with or without a jury. The purpose of an inquest is specified under Coroners Rule 36 of the Coroners Act 1988, referred to above. However, in all contentious deaths – i.e. those raising public interest, as in the case of rail crashes, death in the workplace and in state institutions, for example – a jury is required.[6]

Essentially, there are two types of post-mortem examination (or autopsy): 'one ordered by a coroner, the other a hospital post-mortem agreed upon by the hospital and the next-of-kin.'[7] A coroner post-mortem is a legal require-ment whereas a hospital-based post-mortem is not, but may be requested by the hospital in order to gain a fuller understanding of the patient's illness or treatment. Without the explicit consent of the next-of-kin, it is illegal for hospi-tals to carry out post-mortems.

A post-mortem examination is a medical procedure which consists of three parts, namely: dissection, examination and reporting. It is always performed by a qualified practitioner or a pathologist. After the dead person's body has been dissected, internal organs are removed, weighed and examined visually for any abnormalities. An interim report should be made, immediately after the exami-nation. 'An integral part of a post-mortem examination is the removal of tissue samples [including the taking of fluid samples] and retention of tissue blocks and slides for use in diagnosis, audit and review. [By law the tissue blocks and slides should be returned to the family at the end of the investigation]. This must be explained to the family. Specific consent must be obtained for organs or tissue to be used for research.'[7] Organs such as the brain, because of its delicate and soft structure, have to be removed for laboratory treatment prior to being examined microscopically. The purpose of subjecting the dead body to this procedure is to determine precisely the cause of death, which will be reported to the relatives, clinicians and legal authorities.

Doubts were raised by families in Liverpool regarding the legality of remov-ing and retaining organs at post-mortem. Again, this practice is controlled by legislation. For example, if the coroner decides that a full post-mortem exami-nation is necessary, tissue samples will need to be retained for examination. However, there is no right to retain any parts of the body once the investiga-tion into the cause of death has been completed. The Chief Medical Officer appears to suggest in his report *The Removal, Retention and Use of Human Organs and Tissue from Post-mortem Examination*[8] that the Coroners Rules 1984 (Rule 9) seemed to be ill-understood or knowingly misunderstood by some coroners, as many parents and families had complained about organs being kept. Rule 9 of the Coroners Rules 1984 states that 'a person making a post-mortem examination shall make provision, so far as possible, for the preservation of material which in his opinion bears upon the cause of death, for such period as the coroner thinks fit.'[8] A request for consent for eventual retention of organs or tissue following completion of the coroner's process should be made before the post-mortem is carried out.[7]

Similarly, in the case of the hospital-based post-mortem, removal and retention of tissue or whole organs must be carried out in accordance with the Human Tissue Act 1961. The valid consent of the family or those close to the deceased person must be given before the post-mortem is undertaken to ensure proper compliance with the Act.[7] An ambiguity seems to exist in the Act: 'The Human Tissue Act 1961 provides that the person lawfully in possession of the body of a deceased person may authorise the removal of any part from the body for use for therapeutic purposes or for purposes of medical education or research.' However, the Act goes on to say: '...if, having made such reasonable enquiry as may be practicable, he or she has no reason to believe that the deceased expressed an objection or that the spouse or any surviving relative of the deceased objects to the body being so dealt with.'[7] There will be further discussion on the issue of legal possession of the deceased person. However, my own interpretation of the 1961 Act is that, if consent is not sought and obtained properly from the spouse or any surviving relatives, then the taking and retaining of any part of the deceased person is illegal. Throughout this book we see examples of people complaining that they were not asked, irrespective of how the law might have been interpreted by doctors.

The explanations given so far provide some insight into the complexity of the legal system and allow readers to appreciate the difficulties that many families faced. These families should have been reminded by officials of their rights to raise objections at the time when referrals were made to the coroner or when hospital-based post-mortems were requested. If the rules were not clearly explained or deliberately shielded from them, one could be justified in suggesting that these families in Liverpool and elsewhere might have been deceived. As a result, post-mortems performed by hospital doctors and researchers for reasons of research, education and training could be seen as illegal if they were carried out either without full consent or even without any consent at all.

In the past, the terms 'post-mortem' and 'autopsy' were often used interchangeably. The inconsistent use of terminology by the medical profession could cause further confusion to the public, particularly from the legal perspective. A post-mortem examination requested by the doctors is considered by lay people as a forensic medical investigation as its purpose is to identify the cause of death. Autopsy, on the other hand, could be interpreted as a scientific procedure prescribed by a doctor, a medical scientist in a medical establishment for the purpose of learning, i.e. the study of anatomy or the cause of a disease. In the Shorter Oxford English Dictionary 'autopsy' is described as 'dissection of a dead body, so as to ascertain by actual inspection the cause or seat of disease.'[9] If post-mortems are seen by some doctors as autopsies for the purpose described above, then a supply–demand problem is created since material is needed for study.

Stockpiling is an issue identified by the Royal Liverpool Children's Inquiry team. Readers will remember from Chapter 5 that a huge number of organs, body parts and samples of tissues were held in pathology archives and museums in Liverpool and other parts of the UK.[10] No wonder parents and families challenged the real purpose and necessity of post-mortem examinations in the past. Many examples were brought to the attention of the Retained Organs Commission during 2001 and 2003. A few examples cited here will show families' grievances and their distrust in the post-mortem system.[11]

Example 1: A woman asked at a public meeting: 'My child was born without adrenal glands and he eventually died. The cause of my child's death is therefore known, what then is the purpose of performing a post-mortem?' The post-mortem results in this case might help confirm diagnosis, but to what extent would this new information assist in improving care? Indeed there is no irony in suggesting that perhaps in such a case the doctor knows best. However people are simply no longer automatically prepared to assume this. The next example raises some fundamental issues for the pathologists.

Example 2: 'My daughter had a brain tumour. I gave permission for the brain to be removed. But why take everything else to make sure what the brain did? I don't take electronics out of a machine to find out why the gearbox went down. I acknowledge the need for teaching. But you know how a body works. I know how a gearbox works. I know how a complex machine works with all its electronics. But why do you want the drive shaft? You open the body up. I'll open the machine up. It could have an oil leak or a cable could have gone down or a fuse or a relay. Just by looking at it I can trace it back. Why can't a pathologist do the same by looking at the body with the organs intact? Why does he have to take them all out and stick them in a tray and slice them up?'

Example 3: 'I had a son with a rare condition. They obviously knew what the baby died of because of his apparent [abnormal physical] features. So why did they have to take his brain, his thyroid, his heart, his lungs, spleen and everything else?'

Example 4: 'My son had a brain tumour, but why did they want his toes, his testicles?'

A large proportion of the public was given the impression, wrongly perhaps, that a post-mortem examination was a humane medical procedure. Some had been told that the organs would be put back into the body at the end of the process. The relatives found out that this was not true. A man reported that: 'My wife and I agreed that organs should not be retained... We were promised that [my babies' organs] were put back after the post-mortem. Several years later, we found out that everything was not put back... there were more than one hundred pieces of blocks and slides between two babies... One was two days old, and the other six weeks old. They were both 3lb in weight... nearly the whole of their bodies had been taken out.'[12]

Confusion amongst doctors when putting the law into practice

It seems excusable for the public to be ignorant of the legal position regarding post-mortem examination as it is not its job to know. There is no excuse however for doctors, particularly coroners, not to have a good working knowledge. of the law. More seriously, if coroners had wilfully disobeyed the rules that they were required to follow, then the coroners would be guilty of illegal practice. The practice of coercion as seen in Bristol appeared to be widespread, too. The Redfern report noted that 'there was a lack of precision in the minds of the clinicians as to when a death is strictly reportable to coroner.'[13]

From the informed lay person's point of view (that is to say for people who had reason to look into it), the distinction between hospital post-mortem examination and a post-mortem ordered by a coroner seems to be clear-cut. If lay people can understand the distinction between deaths from natural or known causes and those with no definitive diagnoses, then there is no cause for the hospital doctors to be confused. One could become suspicious of some hospital doctors; they might have an alternative plan for those parents or relatives who showed hesitation in giving consent to a hospital post-mortem, i.e. if they were refused, they were then told it was necessary to report the deaths to the coroner. Such a practice was contrary to the law and was in breach of professional ethics. According to Redfern, 'applying the threat of a coroner's post-mortem examination to obtain consent to a hospital post-mortem examination' was simply illegal.[13]

Was the law a bad regulator of practice or were its defects due to omissions in its terms of reference? The purpose of the Human Tissue Act 1961 was actually 'to make provision with respect to the use of bodies of deceased persons for therapeutic purposes and purposes of medical education and research and with respect to the circumstance in which post-mortem examinations are carried out....' Right away, in that short quotation, there are areas which lack clarity. For example what is the meaning of 'with respect to the circumstance in which post-mortem examinations are carried out'?

So far the technical and legal aspects of post-mortem examination have been discussed but we cannot simply ignore the emotional trauma that has been caused to many by the accepted malpractice of the medical profession and the coroner service. By studying personal accounts of those affected, future practice could hopefully be improved.

Personal Account 1: A baby girl about 20 months old [died] on 5 December 1990 while she was being cuddled. She stopped breathing. [Mother said]: 'I was cuddling her at the time. We phoned for an ambulance which took her to [a local district general hospital]. She was taken away for treatment and we were taken to a waiting room. The doctor came into the waiting room 55 minutes after admission and said: "We are still working on her" but half an hour later, we were told that the girl had died.

'The girl had had two heart operations [about six months before she died] and when she died they [doctors] thought it might have been due to a block or a clot. Although the doctor knew why the girl died why did the doctor ask for a post-mortem? He thought there was a clot in her heart but he wanted to be sure.

'The doctor said they would have to take a sliver of [the girl's lung] at the post-mortem for histology. He said this would determine whether there was a blood clot between the lung and the heart. I asked if they would return all the organs to [the girl's body] after the post-mortem because I knew that the organs were taken out during the post-mortem to be examined. He told me that the organs would be put back.

'I can remember signing the consent form although I cannot remember what it said. I probably did not even read it through before signing it because all I wanted to do was to be with [the girl]. No, I do not remember reading the form. All I was interested in was my daughter. My brain was into holding my child and not wanting to leave the hospital. All I can think of was being with my child and that is all I can visualise now.

'I know that a nurse was also present when I signed the consent form. I can remember but I cannot remember [when] the form [was] being explained to me. I cannot remember anyone told me that I could object to a hospital post-mortem.

'I was informed that there would have to be a post-mortem. No one ever mentioned a coroner's post-mortem to me although a letter from the Trust dated 12 April 2000 states that it was a coroner's post-mortem. I do not know the difference between the two different post-mortems and this was not explained to me. I was not told I could have an independent person present during the post-mortem.

'About [two weeks later] I received a letter from the doctor [who asked for a post-mortem] who said that some further information may be obtained from the histological examination of the lungs. At the time I did not really take the contents of the letter in as it was so close to my daughter's death and I certainly did not realise that this meant that her lungs had been retained. I wrote to the Trust in April 1999 and was told that her heart and lungs had been retained and samples of other tissues. After I wrote again in April 2000, I was told that small pieces of tissue were taken from my daughter's organs and small samples of trachea and lung and that both lungs were retained as well as her brain.

'After the disclosure of Alder Hey, I phoned the Trust again, I was told by the clinical services manager that they had kept my daughter's heart but they had no record of my son who died about 21 years ago when he was two years old.

'I have now finally received the records but they are incomplete. I feel that they are hiding something. I have that feeling which will not go away.'[15]

(Notes were extracted from the Summit evidence documentation. Information in quotes recorded here verbatim.)

Personal Account 2: A full-term apparently healthy baby boy was born about 5 years ago. Unfortunately, two days later he developed an infection in his lower respiratory tract and was taken to the local hospital. The doctors were unable to save him and he died the same day. Fifteen minutes after the boy died, the parents signed a form at the hospital consenting to a post-mortem examination being carried out which also said that 'tissue' might be retained. They had no idea that the word could mean entire organs and it was a decision that would haunt them forever.

Understandably, soon after the death of their baby son the couple did not really know what they were signing. 'We had just lost our baby and couldn't concentrate on anything.' Like hundreds of other parents they were adamant that if they had known the word 'tissue' would be interpreted as meaning major organs, they would never have agreed.

'We were given a leaflet explaining about the post-mortem which said the body would be properly restored for burial. We thought we had buried all of him. Apparently it was a coroner's post-mortem examination which was carried out at the same hospital where the baby was admitted.

'Now, we have been told that virtually all of the boy's organs had been retained in one form or another. The hospital had kept all of his brain, spleen, trachea, larynx, thymus, both lungs, both kidneys, tongue, mesentery, ileo-caecal valve and three vertebrae, part of his heart, liver, rectum, stomach, testes, tissue samples from his skin, bladder, spinal cord, pancreas, pituitary gland and the prostate gland. We are so angry. They stole our son's soul. There was nothing left but an empty shell.'[16]

(The accounts given here are extracts from local newspapers. Every effort has been made to ensure that the details are accurate. Locations will remain anonymous.)

The two family histories above have a number of themes. They serve to remind us of the specific concerns of the public about coroner post-mortems. It has already been said that a large number of families involved did not have any or a great deal of knowledge of either the coroner's or the hospital post-mortem system. Therefore, the families were disadvantaged when being asked for consent for a post-mortem examination. More importantly, those requests were often made at a moment of great emotional vulnerability, as indicated in the second personal account above. The meaning of words doctors use may not be clear and the family's response may not articulate their views. A more detailed discussion on this particular aspect of the consent process will be considered in Chapter 10.

All of us recognise that imparting unpleasant or bad news is an unenviable task for anyone. Having to explain procedures at a time of grief is clearly a tough job. Ideally, doctors and nurses should be trained in this important aspect of medical and nursing care. A close look at these and other case histories suggests that the fundamental complaint is of a lack of openness in talking about post-mortem procedures. Trying to spare parents' feelings in a paternalistic approach may not be the only explanation. It is likely that training had not provided staff with any insight into both the lack of knowledge and the resulting confusion, which was likely to be encountered in dealing with the public over issues involved in post-mortem examination.

Doctors themselves may not have fully understood post-mortem procedures and rules. Families may have been under the impression that they could not refuse a hospital post-mortem examination. If organs were to be kept for further examination, then the responsible doctor should have been more candid in saying so. Fudging such important details about post-mortem examinations could only lead to confusion and create distrust between doctors and relatives. Baseless criticism of medical practitioners does nobody a service. But an intention to deceive, albeit with the best of motives, is difficult to refute in some of the cases.

One might still think: 'Well yes, but I personally would not be bothered by slices of lung being retained. Actually, I cannot see what the problem was if some parts were retained. The doctors were only doing their job.' The pragmatic reader might begin to get closer to a real-life problem when reading that the brain had been taken in the second example. Do you not wonder then whether harvesting organs may be widespread practice? Concern is aroused for decent treatment of the dead; related ethical issues arise that were not previously of interest; both may grow to the point where there is considerable sympathy for the families. One can understand how a grieving parent's feelings are made worse by the procedures and lack of disclosure, and that a sense of grievance is engendered that adds greatly to the existing grief.

The rationale of post-mortems is strongly supported by clinicians and by professional bodies responsible for healthcare. The two accounts above are maybe pursuing the real purpose of post-mortem examinations. But is it really crucial to prove the clinician's diagnosis of cause of death by means of a post-mortem as in the second account? Occlusion caused by a blood clot in the heart or the lung is known to be a fairly common occurrence following major heart surgery. Unfortunately, the complication cannot be prevented when it occurs. It would be reasonable to ask what can be learned from such a post-mortem and whether the purpose was simply to retain the brain and other tissues for subsequent use.

As it is often argued by clinicians that one of the purposes of post-mortem is the desire of relatives to know the actual cause of death, the post-mortem report itself should be submitted to the relatives or their general medical practitioners as a matter of course. GPs often complain that they do not receive post-mortem reports about their patients and feel that it is the responsibility of the hospital and the coroner's office to submit reports to them. The right to know has again been denied to the relatives.[17]

The issue of open communication between hospital authorities and the public has been an ongoing problem according to the National Health Service Ombudsman's reports.[18] Not only that, it has often been said by relatives of patients at Alder Hey and other hospitals that the NHS was deliberately withholding information from them about their relatives' organs.

Callousness of staff has been another common complaint highlighted in the NHS Ombudsman reports.[18] The bad public impression caused by staff attitudes towards organ retention issues is regularly reported at public meetings. NHS staff do not seem to attach any major significance to the way in which people are handled in sensitive and painful situations, as described in the second account above. The lack of respect experienced by many individuals is not something that the health service ought to show.

Certifying and investigating deaths in England, Wales and Northern Ireland – the Shipman Inquiry

Almost by coincidence in January 2000, Dr Harold Shipman was convicted for the murder of 15 of his patients and forging the will of one of them. Harold Shipman's case has further confirmed that there are flaws in the system of reporting deaths to coroners as experienced by many in Bristol, Liverpool and other parts of the UK and further reinforced the notion that van Velzen was not the only aberrant doctor in the medical profession. Trust in the medical profession has been subjected to severe scrutiny as a result.

The Shipman Inquiry was established in January 2001 and Dame Janet Smith was appointed to chair the panel. The terms of reference provided an opportunity for the panel to examine the present systems, together with the conduct of those who had been responsible for operating them in the aftermath of the death of Shipman's victims. The terms of reference covered the actions of the statutory bodies, authorities, other organisations and responsible individuals concerned in the procedures and investigations which followed the deaths of Harold Shipman's patients who died in unlawful and suspicious circumstances.[19]

It was confirmed that Shipman had killed at least 215 of his patients over a period of 24 years. The inquiry's third report stated that it was clear that the arrangements for death and cremation certification and the coronial system which were intended to protect the public against the concealment of homicide had failed to fulfil that purpose. This report further asserted that (a) present post-death procedures show that the families of deceased persons [were] little involved in the process of certification and investigation of a death. The families were not given the consideration they deserve; and (b) the fact that the current arrangements for dealing with the aftermath of a death, especially out of office hours, are unsatisfactory and that there is confusion over what is expected of the police, ambulance service and medical services.[19]

The Shipman Inquiry also indicates that the current system of certifying a death in the community by one single doctor could easily give rise to concealment of crime or wrongdoing. It could also lead to concealment of professional misconduct or clinical errors. The report states that 'Dr Shipman [had] killed more people than any other serial killer yet identified, but we do not know how many other doctors have killed one or more patients. Some such killings have come to light; others may remain hidden. If Shipman was able to kill for almost 24 years before he was discovered, who can say with confidence that there are not other doctors, still unknown, who have killed in the past? Who can say that there will be none in the future?'[19]

The findings of the Shipman Inquiry raised a fundamental question about the public level of trust in the medical profession. Dame Janet Smith said that the system of death investigation and certification 'must seek to protect the public from harm of other kinds and to expose the wrongdoing of others besides an occasional aberrant health professional.'[19] Dame Janet further asserted that the 'discovery of Shipman's crimes has resulted in a substantial loss of public confidence in a system that depends so heavily on the integrity of a single doctor.'[19]

Organ retention scandals throughout the UK, and other reported professional misconduct cases (such as the taking of sexual advantage of patients by gynaecologists and psychiatrists), have put a sharp focus onto the integrity of doctors and the medical profession and the system of professional self-regulation. It would seem that society is not just dealing with one aberrant doctor, be he hospital pathologist or family physician. Dame Janet Smith pointed out that – with systems and safeguards so unsatisfactory – there might well be other situations of which we are totally unaware.

A common theme appears to have emerged. Malpractices can stay hidden for a long period of time. As long as doctors are placed on a pedestal by patients, government, charity organisations, then anxiety will remain and more harm could be done to patients and families.

One can state categorically that murdering patients is unlawful; one can be less categorical that the taking of organs without the knowledge and consent of the deceased's relatives is unlawful. It would appear that the doctors involved could be protected by the inadequacies of the Human Tissue Act 1961. Even if the act of removing and retaining body parts at post-mortem examination is found to be excusable, the traditional image of doctors viewed by the public as god-like figures, endlessly respected by patients, is no longer the case. A parent said during his summing up at the Chief Medical Officer's Summit: 'We all used to treat doctors like gods. We know they are not gods any more. Harold Shipman, James Wisheart, Janardan Dhasmana, Professor van Velzen, Rodney Leadwood, Richard Neil, [are] names that have brought disgrace on the medical profession.'[15]

People were shocked to learn that even one doctor could casually murder his patients; it is so diametrically opposed to the image of medicine as a caring profession requiring long years of training and hard work. It is also disillusioning to learn that doctors can jeopardise their professional careers by acting unprofessionally. Families in Liverpool were shocked by the discovery of Professor van Velzen's practice at Alder Hey, and by the subsequent disclosure that such practices were not unique to Liverpool but widespread throughout the UK.

In the light of the evidence set out in this chapter, It would seem that a more general inquiry should be established to investigate the current system of monitoring of doctors and the management of misdemeanours and mistakes. In order to regain public confidence and to eliminate any further accusations that the medical profession is being allowed to act above the law, the public should be invited to take part in the inquiry. The aim of the inquiry should be to gather evidence of bad systems and of any abuse affecting patients and their relatives in the past, and to give the public the opportunity to put forward their views for future reform.

Death certification and investigation in England, Wales and Northern Ireland – the fundamental review of 2003

In the light of public concerns over post-mortem examination and the system of reporting deaths to coroners as experienced by the public and revealed by the Shipman Inquiry, a fundamental review of death certification and the coroner services was established by the Home Office. The review was chaired by Tom Luce. There were other pressures for a review, such as the Allitt Inquiry into the case of a nurse convicted of murdering four children in her care, the inquiry into the Marchioness and Bowbelle disaster with its disclosure of bizarre post-mortem practices, and of course, the Bristol and Alder Hey inquiries.

The then Home Secretary David Blunkett in his position paper on *Reforming the Coroner and Death Certification Service,* appears to confirm the experiences of the public. Mr Blunkett says: 'The [current] practices do not allow effective performance management or promote consistently high quality; nor do they deliver a cost-effective service across the country [for instance, a bereaved family's experience can vary widely according to where the coroner's investigation takes place].' He further states that 'public inquiries into Bristol Royal

Infirmary and Alder Hey Hospitals, as well as the Marchioness disaster and the murders perpetrated by Harold Shipman, have shown shortcomings throughout the system.'[5] Some families who attended the public meetings of the Retained Organs Commission have also campaigned for a new Coroners Act.

The government intends to retain the coroner system, but is committed to reform. Twelve recommendations have been put forward in the position paper. As a concern of this book is to encourage the public towards a better aware-ness of the system and how it might affect them, the key elements concerning the need of the public will be outlined here. It states in the position paper that the system in future will be 'sensitive to the needs of the bereaved and to provide a high standard of service in what are inevitably difficult circumstances.' The system will allow the family members of the deceased to be more involved in the future as they often provide useful and important information. The more involved role will enable the family to raise concerns more easily. A family charter will be set up giving details of what the family can expect and the family charter will recognise the need to be sensitive towards other faith groups.[5]

The reform of death certification and investigation was long overdue. The wider public expects the system will serve to protect them in the future. The Home Office proposal outlined in 2004 has now been accepted. It is beyond the scope of this chapter to delve further into the precise nature of the Bill, but it is important to emphasise that the public's campaign for change in the coronial system, similar to that of the Liverpool public campaign for change in The Human Tissue Act, has succeeded in gaining a right to challenge coroners.

References

1 Cheung P. Private notes. Retained Organs Commission meeting; 2001: 5th meeting held in Bristol.
2 Cheung P. Private notes. Retained Organs Commission meeting; 2001: 3rd meeting held in Liverpool.
3 Cheung P. Private notes. Retained Organs Commission meeting; 2001: 1st meeting held in London.
4 The Isaacs Inquiry. The Isaacs Report – the investigation of events that followed the death of Cyril Mark Isaacs. London: The Stationery Office; 2003.
5 Home Office. Reforming the coroner and death certification service – a position paper. London: The Stationery Office; 2004: 6–7.
6 Inquest. How the inquest system fails bereaved people. London: Inquest; 2002.
7 Department of Health. Families and post mortems – a code of practice. London: Department of Health Publications; 2003: 3–4.
8 Department of Health. The removal, retention and use of human organs and tissue from post-mortem examination – advice from the Chief Medical Officer. London: The Stationery Office; 2001.
9 Onions CT, editor. *The Shorter Oxford Medical Dictionary*. 3rd ed. London: Guild Publishing.
10 Department of Health. Report of a census of organs and tissues retained by pathol-ogy services in England – conducted in 2000 by the Chief Medical Officer. London: The Stationery Office; 2001.
11 Retained Organs Commission. Minutes of meetings 2001–2003.
12 Retained Organs Commission. Minutes of meeting 2003: 14th meeting held in Sheffield.
13 The Royal Liverpool Children's Inquiry. The Royal Liverpool Children's Inquiry report – summary and recommendations. London: The Stationery Office; 2001: 4.

14   House of Commons. The Human Tissue Act 1961. London: HMSO; 1961.
15   Department of Health: The Chief Medical Officer's Summit – evidence documentation. London: Department of Health; 2001: ref 202.
16   *Nottingham Evening Post*. Body organ outrage: 7 June 2001: 6–7.
17   Berlin A, Wagstaff R, Bhopal R, *et al*. Post-mortem examinations: general practitioners' knowledge, behaviour, and attitudes. *BMJ* 1994: **308**, 1080–81.
18   Cheung P. Phenomenology of Nursing [PhD thesis]. Southampton: Univ. Southampton; 1992.
19   The Shipman Inquiry. The Shipman Inquiry 3rd report – Death certification and the investigation of deaths by coroners. London: The Stationery Office; 2003.

Chapter 7

Ownership of and respect for the body

Validity of the 'no property in a dead body' rule

The medical malpractice of removing and retaining body organs at post-mortem examination for teaching, education and research, arose partly from a long established 19th century 'no property in a dead body' rule when body snatching was commonplace. Because of this rule, body snatching in the 19th century was not a crime. In fact anatomy schools and medical students benefited from the offences committed by Burke and Hare and many similar groups of individuals. Body snatching now would be seen as a totally outrageous and immoral activity as it was in fact in previous centuries.

It is interesting to note the inconsistency of the current legal system. Stealing a body in the present century according to the 19th century law is still not a criminal offence, although a Home Office licence is required for the exhumation of a dead body for forensic investigation purposes. What is the distinction between taking a body from a grave without permission (though we cannot label it as a theft because of the 'no property' rule) and exhumation for an official police investigation? One would suspect if the same rule were applied now in court, the same punishment would be meted out to those found guilty of desecrating a grave with intent to steal a dead body. Obviously the act of stealing a body is socially abhorrent and must be condemned but the law seems powerless as it stands. The same argument could be rehearsed by those who were found to practise the removal of organs from the deceased at post-mortem without consent; hence, relatives who have suffered the consequences of this particular malpractice will not find justice.

No one could possibly imagine the return of the Burke and Hare era as it is considered irrational to commit such an offence. Equally, the removal of organs without consent will hopefully never recur, as promised by the Chief Medical Officer, and the new law is *in situ* to ensure that it will never happen again. But if a case were to be brought to the court, who stands to lose? It would be members of the public who will suffer the anguish experienced by many people in the past. The problem is that the 'no property in a dead body' rule is so entrenched in English and Scottish jurisprudence, that it is almost immutable.[1] It will take another major public outcry to evoke a new Act of Parliament to replace this rule.

As the law stands at present, what, if any, principles are at stake? The Human Tissue Act 2004 specifies that any of the following activities shall be unlawful if done without appropriate consent:

- 'The storage of the body of a deceased person for use for a purpose specified in Schedule 1, other than anatomical examination, shall be lawful if done with appropriate consent.' Schedule 1 specifies that consent is required for 'anatomical examination; determining the cause of death; establishing after death the efficacy of any drug or other treatment administered to him; obtaining scientific or medical information about a living or deceased person which may be relevant to any other person including a future person [the term 'a future person' has not been spelt out in the Act. It could be taken to mean a fetus]; public display; research in connection with disorders, or the functioning, of the human body, and transplantation'

- 'The removal from the body of a deceased person for use for a purpose specified in Schedule 1, of any relevant material [which could include organs, tissue such as blood and urine] which has come from a human body'[2]
- 'The storage for use for a purpose specified in Part 1 of Schedule 1 of any relevant material which has come from a human person.'[2]

If the Human Tissue Act 2004 and the 19th century 'no property in a dead body' rule were to be used in parallel, would there be any ambiguities from the legal point of view? A medical practitioner could have acted unlawfully under the Human Tissue Act 2004 if he were discovered to have removed a body part from the deceased without prior consent of the deceased or where consent was refused by the next-of-kin. However, he/she could be exonerated if the 'no property in a dead body' rule were applied. In that case, is the new Human Tissue Act effective?

If the principle of consent is adjured in this way, the 19th century rule will act against the principle of consent. We should consider here some of the issues around consent. It has been said by McLean and Maher that 'consent is required primarily as a device to ensure that no unlawful interference takes place with the person or the personality of the individual. Traditionally it is deemed to be a means of protecting the right to self-determination which it is held all people have. In other words, rules about the provision of consent are a means of providing for the autonomy of the individual.'[3] If the definition of consent is used in its own right, then one can be assured that the right of the individual will be protected.

In a practical sense, consent does not simply give people a choice about how the body of a fellow human being should be treated after death. Consent also provides the family with an opportunity to exercise altruism in making a gift to the medical profession for education and research, thus benefiting society. Taking without consent means that people are not only deprived of the right to make a choice but that their generosity is usurped. People would resent the fact that their authority to decide has been taken away without leave. From the Liverpool families' point of view, it was perhaps a feeling that they had been robbed of their proprietary right. One could call it a kind of 'death right', exercised by them in trust for the deceased, analogous to the concept of birthright, when the newborn receives gifts from his/her forebears. It is largely symbolic perhaps. Consent by the family remains the key, and in the absence of specific indications left by the deceased, actions such as removal of tissue and organs cannot be undertaken by others who may be in possession of the body at the time of death.

The validity of the 'no property in a dead body' rule can equally be challenged on the basis of ethics and natural law. Muyskens asserts that 'there are two moral principles concerning the rights and duties in respect of the deceased. There is a duty to give decent burial and there must be a denial to anyone of a right of ownership of the dead body for commercial profit, i.e. the body or body parts cannot be sold.'[4] In that case, who has the ultimate right to make decisions for the dead? Does the need to know the cause of death – especially an extended form of that approach – give the clinical point of view precedence over individual rights?

If the 'no property' rule is put against Muyskens' suggested moral imperatives, then how valid is the rule? Further arguments can be put to challenge this. Customarily, the family is responsible for burying the dead; thus by implication, the dead body ultimately belongs to that family, whose members must have the ultimate say in determining whether any parts of the body could be used for teaching, research and therapeutic purposes. The state or any institutions providing service cannot overrule their right. When the Human Tissue Act 1961 remained active, the term 'the person in lawful possession of the dead' took precedence over any public right. It was interpreted by the person in charge of the body that he/she could exercise authority in determining what was to be done with that body until the deceased had been reclaimed by the relatives. Such an erroneous interpretation was also applied by the Department of Health when developing a human hormone for the treatment of retarded growth (*see* Chapter 6).

In effect, it is not unreasonable to define the term 'in lawful possession of the deceased' as the person in charge being given temporary custody of the dead. The responsibility of the custodian is to ensure safe keeping of the subject and to ensure that there is no unreasonable interference to the subject without prior consent. For example, in 1968, the courts in the United States decided that 'the next-of-kin has a right to receive possession of the body immediately after death and in the same condition it was in at the time of death. This right of possession is based upon the principle that each person should have a decent burial and it should be the legal duty of his next-of-kin to provide such.'[5] Although the legal system differs in different countries, ideally the ethical principles upon which legal decisions are determined should be universally applicable. In which case, the legal position stated above should provide the right to anyone in any country to deny permission for the use of organs for therapeutic purposes, teaching and research both now and in the past.

Legal implications of the 'no property' rule for the living

So far the discussion has centred on the legal status of the 'no property' rule in relation to the dead. What are the legal implications for the living if the rule is said to be immutable at present? Currently, it is custom and practice that any form of invasive medical intervention requires explicit written consent from the individual concerned. Without this, it could be judged as a form of assault, from the common sense point of view. The practice of consent will be discussed later in Chapter 10. Currently, advances are being made in cell-line research where human materials such as cells or tissues, including blood, could become someone's intellectual property and could have an enormous monetary value.

The material originally obtained from a human subject with consent could become a patent for the future. Who has the ownership of that patent?

It has been successfully argued, as in Mr Moore's case in California (*see* Chapter 3), that the excised cells or tissues are not owned by the human subject from whom the material was obtained as the characteristics have been altered. One can see the fine line between the 'no property in a dead body' rule and the emergence of a 'no property' rule in a living person. Government departments around the world appear to have the aptitude to make use of loopholes in the legal system. For example, in March 1995, the HTLV-1 (Papua New Guinea T-lymphotropic virus) was patented by the US Department of Health and Human Services, the first human cell-line to be so patented.[6] How relevant is consent in the future if no legal protection is afforded to those who are uninformed?

Of course politicians have the power to bring about legislative change in accord with the relevant social climate. In the light of cell-line development in the US, a new law could be introduced in the near future to replace the 'no property in a dead body' rule to reflect the need to use live cells and tissues for research. This is not too far-fetched as very recently there has been some discussion on the possibility of redefining death. At present, organs would only be removed when the person is diagnosed as brain-dead. But the situation is changing. In June 2006 in Ottawa Hospital in Canada, the first organ transplant in recent history was carried out after a person was declared dead after the heart had stopped. This is referred to as donation after cardiac-death.[7]

The purpose of redefining death could ensure a sufficient supply of organs for transplantation. The counter-argument for such a move is that there has been a case where a person recovered from a car accident having been in a vegetative state for 25 days. One specialist recommended that the life support system be switched off, in which case the heart would have stopped within minutes. If donation after cardiac-death is applied universally, then this person would not have been enjoying her life now despite being wheelchair-bound.[7] There was debate during the passage of the Human Tissue Bill 2003 where some Members of Parliament championed the cause of the opting-out system to combat the problem of organ shortage for transplantation.

Past and present thinking in other EU countries

So what is the past and current thinking of other countries in Europe? In Austria, up to 1982, dissection could take place on anybody who died in a hospital when there was deemed to be general scientific interest. Consent was not required. However, a case in 1978, where a physician was brought to court by the family after splinters of bone were removed without the family's consent, led to a new General Hospital Act. Since then, Austria operates a strict opting-out system where the individual may object to organ removal; the family has no rights in this matter over the deceased relative's body. The new rules state that organ removal may take place unless '...the physicians are in possession of a declaration in which the deceased person, or prior to his death, his legal representative, has expressly refused his consent to organ donation...'[8] In addition, the Austrian physician is neither obliged to seek objections nor to inform the next-of-kin of the intended organ retrieval operation.

The Netherlands does not have a law regarding post-mortem organ removal. The legal rules for organ transplantation, that is consent given via a donor card by either the donor, or his next-of-kin during his lifetime, also apply to the dissection of the corpse. The body can legally be used for whatever purpose. The opting-in law in the Netherlands is supported by the Health Council and the National Council on Public Health.

Similarly, Germany does not have specific legal regulations for organ removal after death; during life, permission for organ removal can be given via a donor card; after death, the next-of-kin may authorise organ removal and retention for transplantation purposes or scientific studies.

In Belgium, until January 1987, post mortem organ retrieval operated by local agreement between the procuring hospitals and the public prosecutor. In February 1987, a new Act stipulated that organ removal from dead patients was allowed unless there were objections from the deceased during his lifetime, or his next-of-kin, after his death.[8]

Are practical issues involved in implementing the opting-out system and what are the implications? This system would require citizens to have expressed a prior wish to dissent. In the absence of this, those who are in lawful possession can decide whatever is appropriate. As a further safeguard, one could also advocate a living-will system in the future, whereby each person would carry a donor card stating his/her expressed wishes. Without this card, one would automatically forfeit the right to raise objections to the manner in which the body might be dealt with after death. If such a system is imposed, then one needs to appoint a legal executor or the next-of-kin to act as proxy, to ensure prior-expressed wishes are carried out by the state. This might be a satisfactory solution so long as the next-of-kin can be found and notified.

In the opting-in system, similar to the current UK system, consent does not apply to minors or to those who are incapacitated. Normally, the parents or guardians of those who are under the age of 16, will agree to express how the body might be treated after death. In England and Wales, it is not permissible for any person to consent on behalf of an incapacitated adult.[1] Therefore in the event of death, the body of anyone incapacitated will be treated either in his own best interest, or in the interest of the public, i.e. either buried or used for medical science.

An insurmountable legal problem

The argument over the ownership of the dead human body goes on, and appears to be a worldwide issue. Recently, a government advisory panel recommended that 'museums in the UK should be allowed to return their collection of human remains to their rightful owners.'[9] Randerson said the US and Australia have already taken significant steps to repatriate human remains.[9] In the UK, some institutions are legally prevented from returning these to descendants in other countries. The expert panel concluded that the desire of indigenous communities to reclaim ancestral remains must take precedence over the rights of scientists to study them.[9] If the expert panel ruling is correct, then the human remains belong to the countries of origin. In that case, could the same rule be applied to judging who has the ownership of the dead body? Does the reluctance to return human remains to the countries of origin have a hidden facet? Would the remains have a commercial value if the objects were to be auctioned? If commercial value could be attached to human remains of historical value, can one then interpret the 'no property' rule established in the English and Scottish systems as invalid, i.e. the human remains so valued belong to their rightful owner?

Using the body for something means that value is attached to the dead body. It has often been said by pathologists, the College of Pathologists and the Department of Health that findings from post-mortem examinations are essential for the understanding and treatment of diseases; therefore the body has a scientific value. In terms of treatment benefit, parts of the body are used for transplantation. In the past, the bodies had a monetary value; bodies were sold to anatomy schools by grave robbers. There was monetary value attached to the removal of pituitary glands, as disclosed by the Isaacs Inquiry.[10] If values are attached to the dead in these situations, is the long established rule of 'no property' still valid?

The problem of ownership of the human body is clearly an insurmountable legal problem as long as the 'no property' rule exists, particularly where the system is flexible and subject to change socially. Perhaps the focus should be on the professional integrity of doctors. At present some may argue that when organs are removed and retained unlawfully, i.e. without explicit consent of the deceased's relatives, then the activity constitutes a form of theft and ought to constitute a legally punishable offence. Similarly, taking living human cells or tissues for the development of cell-line research without the subject being properly informed, should also be regarded as illegal.

Rather than placing trust in the medical profession to control their members and to ensure that the code of conduct is strictly adhered to, some may feel that the criminal law should take over. Those responsible for future legislation should be aware of the possibility that the advantages of a 'stern' approach would need to be balanced against the value of an apparently more 'gentle' approach that would allow doctors to observe and maintain good professional ethical standards. It will be necessary in the future to ensure ethical training of doctors since the law may be insufficient to curb professional misconduct. The medical profession needs to be more self-critical. The legislators also must learn that it is important to legislate thoughtfully and not in haste, to ensure that laws are not contradictory.

It will take time to effect change in human behaviour. Equally, effecting change in the legal system cannot be hurried. In the meantime, guidance might be sought from those families who have had experience of confronting the problem of ownership of their dead relatives.

Most families, if not all, regard post-mortem examination as a form of interference with the person. McLean and Maher's idea of personality referred to earlier in this chapter is an interesting one, in that many families spoke of their deep concern about how their children and relatives looked after death. How essential is it that dead human beings should still preserve their identity and be recognisable? How important are the words used about someone who has ceased to be a living being? Does it mean that by referring to the deceased person as the 'corpse' or 'the body', this actually alters the nature of the person's identity? How far should those qualities and impressions that are collectively referred to as our personality be preserved and protected not only in life but in death also? How much external interference is permissible? Is there any cultural, ethical or faith view that would not regard as abhorrent any form of unnecessary interference resulting in disfigurement? What seems a trite line of thinking becomes more vital when it is remembered that burial was allowed to take place in at least one case despite the retention elsewhere of the head. Given the element of concealment involved, the retention of a heart, brain, eye, hand, etc. of a dead person is surely an insult both to the living and the dead.

Dwelling on these thoughts of disfigurement might seem irrational and exaggerated to some. Just as attitudes to death can vary greatly so can attitudes to the dead body. Experience of death of others also of course varies greatly between individuals and eras, i.e. between wartime and peace, and between times of epidemic disease and the generally better medical conditions of modern life. In his book entitled *Theology, Death and Dying* Anderson classifies death as a posthumous experience.[11] Presumably he means that no one in life can experience death. Clearly attitudes to the human body in the time between death and burial or cremation require empathy, and this may be difficult since our experience is limited. Therefore it seems sensible that medical education and ethical guidelines should encourage the doctor to be respectful to the dead body even when the need for research or forensic investigation provides the motive for interference.

The question of ownership of the human body remains unresolved, which is an important concern for all of us. 'Who has the right to remove and retain my son's or daughter's or my relative's organs?' is one of the questions often raised by members of the public who were the subjects of a medical malpractice. Based on findings of various Inquiries one can understand the basis of their question. On the other hand, there are others both inside and outside the medical profession who would simply say: 'What is the fuss about?'

This opinion was often heard in informal discussion at conferences and in NHS hospital trust boardrooms. A Roman Catholic priest said, in an informal conversation about 5 five years ago when the Alder Hey events hit the headlines that he just could not see 'what the fuss was about'. He felt he personally was not bothered one way or another how his body would be treated after death. Perhaps his theist stance transcends the issues of consent and the value attached to the human body for transplant surgery or for teaching and research. Those who do not have the wisdom of the priest will see the expression at best as insensitive and at worst as insulting.

Those of us who were detached from organ retention malpractice simply did not comprehend the significance of the indignity of being lied to by doctors and hospital managers about where children's organs were kept, and did not understand what it meant not knowing whether their children had been buried intact; did not understand what it felt like having to bury their children more than once due to misinformation and poor cataloguing of retained organs in the past; and failed to share the sense of injustice that no one was held accountable for the wrongdoing.

One also needs to consider the importance of medical progress since transplant surgery is now a normal practice. The shortage of donor organs is real. Perhaps there might be a strong case to support research on the manufacturing of autograft from one's own stem cells for organ transplantation. It will avoid any ambiguous discussions over ownership or consensual issues. It will allow medical progress without ethical and legal hindrances. It is difficult of course to ascertain without further research how people from different cultures would react to the notion of using organs obtained from reproductive cloning in medical practice. This is another 'brave new world' which might alter the fundamental values one holds in a human society.

References

1 Mason K, Laurie G. Consent or property? Dealing with the body and its parts in the shadow of Bristol and Alder Hey. *Modern Law Review* 2001; **64**(5): 710–729.

2 Human Tissue Act 2004: Elizabeth II: Chapter 30. London: The Stationery Office; 2004.

3 McLean S, Maher G. *Medicine, Morals and the Law*. Aldershot: Gower; 1983: 79.

4 Muysken JL. An alternative policy for obtaining cadaver organs. In: *Philosophy and Public Affairs* reader. New Haven: Yale University Press; 1970.

5 Sander D, Dukeminier J, Jr. Medical advance and legal lag: Hemodialysis and kidney transplantation. *UCLA: Law Review*; 1968: **15**: 402.

6 Rifkin J. *The Biotech Century*. New York: Penguin Putman; 1998.

7 Nowak R. Not brain-dead, but ripe for transplant – a drive to increase the number of organs taken before they become unusable is dividing the medical world. *New Sci.* 2006; **191**(2563): 6–7.

8 Kokkedee W. Kidney procurement policies in the Eurotransplant region. 'Opting in' versus 'opting out'. *Soc Sci Med* 1992; **35**(2): 177–82.

9 Randerson J. Experts squabble over ancient bones. *New Sci.* 2003; **180** (2421): 9.

10 The Isaacs Inquiry. The Isaacs Report – the investigation of events that followed the death of Cyril Mark Isaacs. London: The Stationery Office; 2003.

11 Anderson RS. *Theology, Death and Dying*. Oxford: Blackwell; 1986.

Chapter 8

Natural law and medical research

Natural law and its relevance

The subject of natural law is important for human society as it prescribes some general precepts that will enable people to distinguish sound from unsound thinking, separate those acts that are reasonable from those that are unreasonable. It provides a set of practical moral standards upon which everyone should operate. It helps people to decide ways of acting that are morally right or morally wrong. The principles of natural law apply to almost every aspect of human life including the drive for self-preservation, the pursuit of knowledge, aesthetic experience, practical reasonableness (defined as ability to use intelligence to bring about effective action), the pursuit of friendship and the practice of religion.[1] If the principles of natural law apply to all citizens, then how relevant is natural law to medical research in general and, more specifically, to the use of the human body for research, including the use of cells, tissues, for new medical developments?

The pursuit of knowledge is an important aspect of medical practice and research, as doctors and scientists are required to keep abreast of advancements in order to effect improvements in standards of care. Some are more concerned with the discovery of new theories and practice. The pursuit of knowledge and understanding is regarded as a basic human good so that one is able to make correct judgements. Of course, there is the question of whether one should seek to improve one's knowledge just for the sake of knowing. Doctors at Alder Hey have been criticised for the habit of collecting children's eyes for the sake of collecting as an end in itself. Was there a need for doctors to violate basic human values for the sake of research and at the expense of basic human values by inflicting pain on others?

Integrity is a form of practical intelligence, according to St Thomas Aquinas,[2] which needs to be cultivated. From Aquinas' point of view, no one can be morally upright if he/she has not grasped (a) the first principle of practical reasoning and (b) practical reasonableness which is not a speculative quality, but the ability to apply one's intelligence to particular commitments, projects or action, thus enriching human existence.

St Thomas Aquinas sees the practice of religion as a form of basic human good. However, he does not see religion purely from the theoretical perspective but also as a way to respond to specific problems in human society. The Catechism of the Catholic Church states that 'the divine and natural law [as opposed to civil law] shows man the way to follow so as to practise the good and attain his end. The natural law expresses the original moral sense which enables man to discern by reason the good and evil, the truth and the lie.'[3] The emphasis of the Catholic Church is on man's ability to exercise reason; this allows us to distinguish between good and evil. It seems unlikely that other religious faiths would dissent from such a view.

Adopting the principles of natural law in medical research would mean that researchers must act reasonably in applying science in the laboratory and in clinical settings. Researchers are expected to exercise integrity when human subjects, both living and dead, are used for their studies. Scientists and researchers must pay due regard to individuals' religious beliefs, customs and practices. Respect for religious practice may not seem immediately relevant in the field of medical research, but if we re-examine some of the non-compliance issues discussed in Chapter 5, the significance of this basic rule would become apparent.

Violation of natural law and post-mortem

Natural law is not faith-specific. It is even more important therefore to observe such rules in a multi-cultural and not completely western orientated secular society. It would be difficult to find many people who would disagree with the principle that the human body must be treated with reverence. One might quibble with the word reverence, but it is defined in the dictionary as being deeply respectful. At the Chief Medical Officer's Summit following the publication of the Redfern Report, in which representatives from various faith groups attended and gave evidence, they seemed to share the commonly held value of paying respect to the dead.

The Summit was attended by a good number of the Jewish community whose relatives' organs had been taken without their knowledge and discarded. 'They are still suffering and their lives are blighted on a daily basis.'[4] The Registrar of the London Beth Din (which is the Court of the Chief Rabbi) points out that 'post-mortem examinations are to be avoided whenever possible, not only because they cause a delay in burial but also because they constitute in Jewish law a violation of the dignity of the dead body.'[4] On behalf of the Jewish community, the Registrar recommended that a non-invasive procedure, such as MRI (magnetic resonance imaging), would be more appropriate if post-mortem were required. He further considered it vital that proper time be given to relatives to reflect on whether or not to consent to post-mortem, and if in doubt, opportunity should be given to them to discuss their decision with their religious advisers.[4]

A retired cardiothoracic surgeon, representing the Muslim Council of Britain and the Muslim Doctors and Dentists Association, reiterated his dismay and serious concern at the treatment given to dead children at Alder Hey hospital. He regarded the practice up to 1999 as 'contrary to the law of common humanity and it is a careless disregard of the pains and suffering of families involved. Such practice must be challenged to ensure that further suffering will not fall upon other families in the future.'[4] The Muslim Council of Britain and the Muslim Doctors and Dentists Association asserted that 'we have got great regard and respect for the dead body. In many ways our ideas are very similar to Christians, Hindus and even Sikhs from my limited knowledge on the subject. Any hurt or denigration of the dead body, however important in terms of scientific progress, is unacceptable.'[4] Therefore, in his view, these attitudes towards the dead person are universally held, irrespective of faith.

During the period when complaints about organ retention were being investigated, a member of the public presented his personal experience at one of the public meetings, which would serve to remind clinicians and researchers of the importance of having a good understanding of both religious beliefs and attitudes of different faiths, and the necessity of observing these practices.

'In 1991, my wife, at just turned 62, had what is called a minor operation to ease the pain in her right arm in a hospital here. Within weeks, she suffered a subclavian thrombosis and lost the use of her left side of her body, the left arm and leg. She was moved from hospital to a rehabilitation ward.

'After about four months, they told me I had to take her home as there was nothing they could do for her...

'I took her home and I had to give up work to look after her. I learned the ropes to keep her alive. Until the final 24 hours she was in full possession of her mental faculty though her body was paralysed...

'My wife was a devout Hindu. My daughter was brought up in England and she hardly knew anything about Hindu traditions and religious requirements, so somewhere two doctors prevailed upon her and got her to sign a consent form to carry out a post-mortem, without my knowledge because I was very distraught... Eventually the post mortem was carried out, all her organs from her body were removed without us being told...I cremated her by Hindu traditions, not the way it should have been as there was nothing inside her...I was in danger being [of being] excommunicated by my own society...

'I got a letter from the chair of the hospital trust expressing their sympathy and offering £750 for the distress I have suffered. My family, myself, my two grandchildren were devastated by this. £750 for our traditions.'[5]

Violation of religious law was the subject of the public inquiry that was briefly described in Chapter 5. Those who practise Judaism see post-mortem examination as an irreverent interference with the human body. In the Isaacs' situation, the cause of death was known and the investigating team was told by Mr Isaacs' widow that Jewish Law forbade post-mortem. However, a post-mortem was carried out on 27 February 1987, less than twenty-four hours after the death of Mr Isaacs. His family was unaware that his brain had been inappropriately retained for research at Manchester University.[6] On 5 April 2000, Mr Isaacs' widow found that an undated letter from the Department of Psychiatry at Manchester University was sent to Mr Isaacs' GP, informing him that the 'university had collected samples of Mr Isaacs' brain....'[6] Mrs Isaacs and her family felt that this was an affront to Mr Isaacs' religious beliefs and those of his family.

It is not at all certain how many people have been subject to the same treatment. To help future professionals and researchers avoid further alienation from respective faith groups, an attempt is made here to summarise faith issues, as a guide to good practice. It is hoped that readers will continue to acquire knowledge and understanding in this field so that people's rights are respected. I am making a general assumption here about Christianity; that the basic doctrinal principles are applicable to all denominations within the Christian church including Methodist, Wesleyan, Presbyterian, etc. which diversified from within the Church of England.

As shown in Table 8.1, those who practise traditional Jewish Laws (Halacha) would see post-mortem examination in most cases as a form of desecration, being disrespectful, irrelevant and an outrageous treatment of the dead. In 1737, Rabbi Jacob Emden rejected the notion of gaining benefit from the study of the dead. However, Rabbi Emden's view could now be set aside. Islam sees the body as sacred and belonging to God; it strongly opposes post-mortem. Some authoritative Jewish and Islamic writers would suggest that continuing dialogue on the subject of autopsy would lead to growth and diversity in the body of opinion.[7,14]

Although Judaism and Islam oppose unnecessary interference with the body, there are no absolute rules about organ donation and organ transplantation. Most faith groups would see organ donation as a gift, and therefore a meritorious act. However, all faith groups emphasise the importance of respect and dignity, which are perceived as rules of natural law. Most humanists outside religious denominations would respect these views and practices, because tolerance is usually a principle of humanist ethics.

There is no clear statement from many of the Christian denominations on post-mortem examination as a scientific procedure and as a form of study. However, the Plymouth Brethren are deeply concerned about 'unnecessary and uncontrolled interference with our bodies. Since 1978 we have been consistently asking the government to recognise Christian conscience in providing protection for our bodies in these circumstances. We respect government as being of God for there is no power without God: the powers that be are ordained of God.'[17]

No previous research has been carried out to investigate the attitudes of Jewish, Islamic and Christian faiths towards the use of stem cells for treatment and research. According to the current state of knowledge, one can assume support for using embryonic stem cells in the manufacture of whole organs for transplantation, as the intention is to save life. Drug trials, particularly for those religions that proscribe the use of medication in any form, would not be permitted. Most Christian denominations would support any form of therapeutic programme, provided the integrity of the recipient is protected.

Respect for the dead

Members of the public have questions about the basic rights of users in a health service; the authority of the medical profession, the authority of the individual to consent or object to post-mortem examination, the right to object to the removal and retention of body organs at post-mortem examination, the consequences of misuse of authority by the medical profession. They also critically examine some basic human values such as openness and transparency in personal interaction and in communication, decency and respect for the living and the dead. They also emphasise respect for human rights within post-mortem examination and pathology practice, especially respect for particular religious beliefs and faith practices.

Not all families in Liverpool, Bristol and around the country expressed any fervent religious belief, but all members of the public believed that children and adults should be buried intact. Many families believed that organs were 'put back' into the bodies of their relatives after post-mortem examination before

Table 8.1 The table summarises some of the documentary evidence of three faith groups regarding autopsy, organ retention and organ donation.

Religion	Funeral rite	Autopsy	Organ retention	Organ donation
Christianity Roman Catholic and Church of England	*Burial or cremation; *The Roman Catholic church permits cremation provided that it does not demonstrate a denial of faith in the resurrection of the body[3]	Papal ban on human dissection was lifted in 1556. Currently, post-mortem not proscribed. In fact, autopsies can be morally permitted for legal inquests or scientific research[3]	No official pronouncement against using organs for teaching, education and research but the bodies of the dead must be treated with respect in faith and hope of the Resurrection[3]	No official directives from all churches; subject to individual conscience. The free gift of organs after death is legitimate and meritorious[3]
Judaism	Burial	*Traditional Jewish Laws (Halacha) opposes post-mortem; *Rabbi Jacob Emden in 1737 stated that no benefit should derive from dead bodies;[7] *Rabbi Jacob Emden's opinion could be overlooked; *Prohibition not found in Jewish Laws or regulations in the Bible or post Bible sources such as Talmud *Post-mortem as a desecration has no basis in Jewish legal sources; *some would support autopsy if it is done to increase medical knowledge[9] or to assist in relieving suffering[10]	Organs used for research not permitted unless it is related to a rare specific condition[8]	*Not against organ transplantation. *Organs used for transplant in Jewish Law must be taken while respiration and circulation is ongoing profused by external means when brain is certified dead. Pikuach Nefesh specifies the obligation is to save human life[8]
Islam	The dead must be buried, never cremated	*Body is sacred and belongs to God, therefore, post-mortem not permitted[11] *against dissection for learning and study of anatomy[12,13] *Neither Koran nor Hadith addresses the issue of autopsy[14,15] *disfigurement of the dead forbidden[7] * Fatawa supports the notion of learning if benefits of autopsies outweigh the drawbacks and if medical students and physicians can learn from them	* As removal of organs and brains involves breaking of bones – Muslims believe that breaking the bones of a dead person is like breaking the love of a living person[15,16] This rule could be relaxed in certain circumstances, e.g. suspect of murder	Prolongation of life by artificial means is strongly disapproved of unless there was evidence that a reasonable quality of life would result[12]

burial and cremation. Their belief was unfounded, as events in Alder Hey, Bristol, and many other locations revealed. Those who were followers of Christianity also believed that bodily mutilation after death constituted an affront to humanity and Christian belief. Strong support and respect should be given to those whose religious beliefs lead to objection to the principle of post-mortem. Their campaign against unnecessary interference with the human body after death is also supported by Article 9 of the Human Rights Act, 1998, which calls upon government to recognise the right to freedom of thought, conscience and religion.

One of the questions often asked by families concerns the disposal of their relatives' organs. How was my child's brain disposed of? Were the organs incinerated? Parents often said 'we thought we had buried them whole. It is not possible to imagine that our children were buried without their hearts or brains.' Brains and hearts are major organs of the human body, and they appear to have a special meaning attached to them. For example, one of the parents at the CMO Summit was asked how organ retention had affected her. She said: 'I believe that they [children] went to heaven but at the same time the heart is where you love from, the bit that makes you your sole [soul]. Your soul is supposed to go to heaven with you. My child was robbed and we were robbed, too. We tried to do our best for her and I feel we let her down.'[4]

Some people may have the mythic notion that the heart represents love and passion, and that the brain, as the centre of imagination, the mind or the psyche, controls being. For some religious people, the brain represents the soul. Those readers who can remember the infancy of heart transplantation surgery will recall how potential recipients of a new heart wondered whether their psychological and emotional profiles would change, if the donor heart were from a person of the opposite sex. I think one lesson that has been learnt from Alder Hey and similar events, is that there is widespread unease about burial of bodies without major organs. For the religious, faith may influence their reaction to post-mortem procedures in a variety of ways, although there is not necessarily unanimity of interpretation within each faith or church.

Burial or cremation is regarded by most, if not all, as the final goodbye – it's the last respect due to the dead. Exhumation, perceived as a threat to this final act of respect, has always been a practice only allowed in law in exceptional circumstances. Equally, most of us could not contemplate the possibility of having to bury our dead more than once. The very name of the family support group in Liverpool – PITY II (Parents who have Interred their Young Twice) – draws attention to the pain and grief caused by the actions of the medical profession.

In the debate over the new Human Tissue Bill 2003, some MPs spoke of the additional grief and suffering faced by families who had to bury their relatives' remains again and again. Martyn Jones, MP for Clwyd South, told of a particular case in his constituency: '...a family in my constituency whose daughter Kayleigh was subject to the problem of Alder Hey. They had three lots of organs returned to them, which has made them distraught over 11 years.'[18] Another MP representing Belfast South recounted another situation where the family was subjected to similar treatment by the medical profession. He said: 'People gave permission on certain organs, but no more. However, that was not accepted and later on they were horrified to discover not only that things had been done against their wishes, but that the residue was sent back to them separately, leading to three separate interments.'[18]

On another occasion, the MP representing Liverpool West Derby, said: 'Following inquiries into the events at Alder Hey, however, it became apparent, as my Right Hon. Friend, the Member for Holborn and St Pancras (Mr Dobson) said, that the storage of human organs and tissue without consent was widespread. Both the hospital and university authorities – they have not been mentioned specifically in the debate so far – were culpable. ... Parents were told at the time of bereavement that all organs had been returned to the bodies. That was untrue. The situation was horrendous, and as has been said, in some cases the bereaved parents had to endure multiple funerals. Even where consent was given, the parents had no idea that it meant the extraction of all organs and that what they were burying were the mere shells of their loved ones.'[19]

The MP for South Cambridgeshire's contribution was: 'It was not due only to the events at Alder Hey and Bristol that the retention of organs gave rise to considerable distress. Many Members from all parts of the country will share my experience in my constituency, and will have met families of those whose relatives' organs or tissue were retained without consent or, in some instances, directly contrary to their expressed wishes. One of my constituents told me of the loss of their son in a road traffic accident in 1984. At the time, they did not wish any of his organs to be retained after the coroner's post-mortem and were assured by the undertaker that that was not the case and their son had been buried intact. Members will thus appreciate the distress when they made inquiries at the time of the press reports on the Alder Hey findings and found that Addenbrooke's Hospital, in my constituency, had in fact retained their son's appendix. After systematic collection and examination of the hospital records...the family found that not only had their son's appendix been retained, but also his thymus. On successive occasions, many years later, they had to arrange further interment of their son's remains.'[18]

The MP for Sutton and Cheam further raised the issue of respect for the dead when the Human Tissue Bill 2003 was being debated in January 2004. The part of the transcript of the CMO Summit he cited sums up the feelings of the parents who spoke on that day, and, generally the feelings of those of the public who were not present at the Summit. The transcription states: 'It almost was – I mean, if I could just use an analogy, it was almost like scrap cars being taken to a scrapyard. The cars were dismantled, the alternators were taken out, the batteries were taken out, put on a shelf, then when somebody comes along and wants one of those parts they pay for it. In the case of our children, they were disassembled completely. The organs were stored, never used.'[20]

To do good in all circumstances

As discussed earlier in this chapter, one of the purposes of natural law is to guide individual actions in ordinary circumstances. Knowledge, understanding, the curiosity to find out more together with personal integrity, enhance intelligent actions that will uphold basic human values such as honesty, decency, respect. There is a tendency for those in authority in the health service, to disparage those whom they serve. We have heard it said a few years ago by a group of scientists in Cambridge referring to their latest innovation, that the public need not know what was being done and in any case, would not understand it. We have also seen examples where some professions chose to apply the technique of coercion when seeking consent for post-mortem examinations. According to Aristotle 'coercion is for the recalcitrance of the selfish, the brutish whose unprincipled egocentricity can be moderated by a direct threat to self-interest.'[21]

Medical research is governed by ethical and civil rules. The purpose of these rules is to provide authority in directing individual behaviour and to give legal validity to all those who work within that community. Therefore, everyone must comply with these laws. Thus for the common good of the community, sanctions or penalties as appropriate, must be applied to those who flout the rules. According to natural law, punishments and legal sanctions serve to avoid injustice and bring about fairness in the system. Having a system in place encourages professionals and researchers to avoid the type of recklessness and negligence seen in many instances in recent years.

Other natural law principles such as duty, respect for others' rights, (e.g. the right to object, the upholding of truth), are also relevant to medical research. These principles should apply both to the living and the dead. There are many examples in previous chapters of people who, in the name of medical research, have been denied the right to information necessary for making informed choices, and the right to object to disrespectful treatment to the dead. Natural law serves to remind all those who engage in medical research to follow their basic human instinct to do good in all circumstances.

References

1   Finnis J. *Natural Law And Natural Rights.* Oxford: Clarendon Press; 1980.
2   Aquinas T, Kenny A, editors. *A Collection Of Critical Essays.* London: Macmillan; 1969.
3   Catechism of the Catholic Church. London: Geoffrey Chapman; 1998: 426–7. Reproduced by kind permission of Continuum of International Publishing Group.
4   Department of Health. The Chief Medical Officer's Summit – proceedings. Held at Queen Elizabeth II Conference Centre; 2001 January 11- computer-aided transcription by Harry Counsell and Co. London. 2001 London: Department of Health: 11–13.
5   NHS Retained Organs Commission. Minutes of 12th meeting 2002; Newcastle-upon-Tyne.
6   The Isaacs Inquiry. The Isaacs Report – the investigation of events that followed the death of Cyril Mark Isaacs. London: The Stationery Office; 2003.
7   Geller SA. Religious attitudes and the autopsy. *Arch Pathol Lab Med* 1984; **108**: 494–6.
8   Beth Israel Congregation. Organ donation in Jewish Law – summary of discussion at Beth Israel; 22 June 1996. Beth Israel Men's Club.
9   Maslin SJ, editor. *Gates of Mitzvah: a guide to the Jewish life cycle.* New York: CCAR Press; 1987: 140–2.
10 Stern C, editor. *On the doorposts of your house.* New York: CCAR Press; 1994: 33.
11 Darsh SM. *Islamic health rules.* London: TAHA; 1986.
12 Radman F. *Health and medicine in the Islamic tradition.* New York: Crossroad; 1987.
13 Al-Sijistani, Sulayman AD. Cited in AR Gartrad. Muslim customs surrounding death, bereavement, postmortem examinations and organ transplants. *BMJ* 1994; **309**: 521–3.
14 Rispler-Chaim V. The ethics of postmortem examination in contemporary Islam. *J Med Ethics* 1993; **19**:164–8.
15 Gatrad AR. Muslim customs surrounding death, bereavement, postmortem examinations, and organ transplant. *BMJ* 1994; **309**: 521–3.

16 Ghanem I. Permission for performing an autopsy: the pitfalls under Islamic law. *Med Sci Law* 1988; **28**: 241–2.

17 Taylor S, Robertson B. *Post-mortem examinations and Christian conscience* (campaign leaflet). Andover and Oxford: Taylor & Robertson; 2002.

18 Great Britain. House of Commons. Hansard. Official Report. 2004; **416(22)**: 985.

19 Great Britain. House of Commons. Hansard. Official Report. 2004; **416(22)**: 1019–1020.

20 Ibid. **416(22)**:1006.

21 Radice B, Baldick R, editors. *Aristotle – Ethics*. London: Penguin Books; 1951.

Chapter 9

Issues of public trust

Erosion of public trust

The issue of professional trust is an interesting one, as lay people, defined as anyone who is not a member of a particular profession under discussion, seldom question the judgement of a qualified person. Each profession is endowed, almost without question, with a generous gift from the public called trust, which is taken for granted most of the time. The trust attached to each profession is perhaps associated with the recognition that training is involved, and that there are specific requirements that each professional has to fulfil, e.g. examinations, prior to their being allowed to practise. In addition, each profession has its own code of conduct that all members must observe. The purpose of the code is to ensure, at least in theory, that the interests of the public are protected.

The trust given to the profession is also passed on to individual practitioners, by virtue of their registration with their own professional body. Once registered, each practitioner becomes an ambassador of that profession. The image of each professional group is a collective one, but the image can be damaged by a group, or groups, of practitioners who fail to comply with the professional rules or laws that govern their particular sphere. There are safeguards, however, to ensure that the image of each profession is upheld by all members at all times. If a registrant is proved negligent, then he/she can be removed from that professional register by their professional body.

The General Medical Council (GMC), the main regulatory body for the medical profession in the UK, was established by Act of Parliament in 1858. The principal functions of the GMC are:

- to oversee medical education and the examinations leading to qualification
- the registration of qualified medical practitioners and the publication of the Medical Register
- the removal of registrants convicted of felony
- the prosecution of unqualified practitioners who had presented themselves as licensed
- the publication of a British pharmacopoeia.[1]

The other purpose of professional regulation which is not mentioned in any official document is to ensure that the public has a proper channel through which to challenge the standards and moral behaviour of professionals.

There are procedures laid down for complaints to be reported and investigated. For example, NHS users can raise their complaints about individual practitioners with their local health trust, and the complaints will be investigated. If complainants are not satisfied with the result of the local investigation, they can have recourse to an appropriate arbitration authority, e.g. education matters can be referred to Ofsted. In the NHS, the Parliamentary and Health Service Ombudsman acts as the arbitrator for any unsolved complaints raised by the public about healthcare and behaviour of all health staff. Alternatively, members of the public can report misdemeanours, or malpractice, directly to the professional regulatory body such as the General Medical Council (GMC), or the Nursing and Midwifery Council (NMC), for investigation.

How much confidence does the public have in professional self-regulation? There are many incidents from the past which raise doubts about the judgement of the professional body; in some cases the judgement passed upon the individuals appears unclear to the complainants, and often there are no explanations given as to why certain decisions are made. The public needs to know the criteria upon which judgement is made, in every situation. The process of investigating complaints or malpractice must be open and transparent. There should be opportunities for the public to sit in on disciplinary cases, so they can understand the issues raised and discussed by both sides. There should be provision for the public to examine documentary evidence in retrospect.

Professor van Velzen was referred to the GMC by the Chief Medical Officer for professional misconduct. He was struck off the medical register. There were other doctors involved in the malpractice at Alder Hey, who were considered complicit in a widespread malpractice of removing and retaining organs without consent. They therefore should also have been referred to the GMC for investigation. The public is confused about why only van Velzen was reported to the GMC. There is a wider issue of justice here, as many other doctors are also involved throughout the UK, but why was only one group of doctors, in one particular location, examined?

The public is also looking for unity of agreement between the professional regulatory authority and the law. There are cases where the judgement between the two is contradictory. Roy Meadow, as an expert witness, gave evidence in court which resulted in a miscarriage of justice. He was found guilty of professional misconduct and struck off by the General Medical Council. Meadow appealed against the GMC's decision; Mr Justice Collins upheld Meadow's appeal, stating that this doctor made the mistake of misunderstanding and misinterpreting the statistics.

The discrepancy in judgement between the GMC and the court is clearly gross. This would be an interesting case for further public investigation. In the light of this particular case, there is a requirement for the GMC to consider whether the legal advice given to them, was sound. One might suspect that the 'club culture' ethos could influence the final proceedings in the appeal procedures. In a situation like this, the public is confused; trust in the whole medical profession is eroded as the public questions the efficiency of the professional regulatory machinery.

In the case of Harold Shipman, how was it possible for the professional body to allow his criminal practices to continue for over 20 years, without being discovered? How efficient is the system in monitoring general practitioners? In the light of the van Velzen case, trust should not be an automatic gift. There needs to be proof that each practitioner, and the profession as a whole, is trustworthy. The medical profession needs to conduct a thorough self-assessment of its philosophy and code of conduct, as well as the effectiveness of self-regulation. There have been occasions in the past 20 years where the medical regulatory framework has been revised because of a series of internal and external problems, which had caused crises of confidence in the GMC, and in the profession as whole.[1,2,3,4,5] Revising the professional code of conduct or the regulatory framework in response to crises, could be seen as a 'knee-jerk' reaction, which does not inspire public confidence in the ability of the profession to maintain standards.

The crisis management approach to professional standards and ethics hardly inspires confidence, as it suggests that there were serious flaws in thinking within the medical profession. In the light of the recent events, one wonders whether professional self-regulation is the appropriate way forward for medicine. In addition, sections of the public are aware that self-regulation does not work for medicine. The public will give the profession more credence if it admits that the practice of medicine and its associated activities should be regulated by a different method, e.g. inspection by a team comprising a range of professionals and lay people, and appointed by the Public Appointments Commission. No doubt some members of the profession will canvass against such a radical shift. The public might need to take part in the longer-term debate.

There is not an agreed system for the regulation of medical research, though there are a number of gatekeepers involved in the process of determining whether proposals and research activities adhere to ethical guidelines, as previously discussed in Chapter 3 of this book. The purpose of the Nuremberg Code, Declaration of Helsinki, etc is to ensure that no harm will be done to human subjects who have been enrolled into specific research programmes. However, these codes are not legally binding. One could choose to ignore them.

We have discussed some of the issues surrounding the gatekeepers in research and ethics approval. The prime function is to ensure that the conduct of individual research does not contravene guidelines, and that methods are appropriately employed. At present, once approval is given, the researchers are free to conduct their research activities without any subsequent monitoring by the local research ethics committees (LRECs), if the research is mono-centred, or from the Central Office for Research Ethics Committee (COREC). The R&D committees in all health trusts currently provide the initial screening and approval process. In theory, the system should be sufficiently robust to highlight unethical practices, but in reality it does not work with good effect, as reported in the findings of the Isaacs Report.

It is worth considering this case in order to further identification of issues concerning the current research and ethics approval procedures of any LRECs.

'In seeking research funds for the programme, the consent of the relatives was emphasised in the applications to funding bodies and in protocols to the local ethics committees. Ethics committees and research funding bodies were not told that most of the brains collected in the programme were from coroners' cases. [It is worth noting that coroners are not authorised by law to retain body parts without explicit consent from the relatives].

'Applications to ethics committees were made by the [principal researcher] on behalf of the joint programme. Although the ethics committees had not been told about collection of brains from coroners' cases, letters sent to general practitioners requesting medical details of their deceased patients stated that the studies had ethical approval. The GMC guidance, current at the time, was that information should only be released for research that had ethical approval. The letters also misinformed general practitioners by referring to "brain samples", where, in most cases, the research team had the whole brain.

'The collection of brains of long-stay patients in mental hospitals who had no relatives was, in one letter, encouraged in the following terms: "often chronic patients don't have next-of-kin, in which case there is no difficulty." This disregards the need for consent from those responsible for vulnerable patients who had no one else to speak for them.'[4]

Assuming that doctors had not intended to tell lies to the relatives and to research ethics committees in order to obtain funding for the research, what went wrong? Although the intention of the principal researcher may have been good, the means used to obtain funds and human specimens belie that assumption. The research team was shown to have avoided fundamental ethical principles, and to have demonstrated overt disobedience to standards of professional conduct. Would conduct have been the same, worse or better, with the imposition of the scrutiny of a committee on the researchers? A better question is: how can, or should, a committee avoid such a disregard of its sanctions?

As a rule, all documents regarding consent, including an information sheet outlining the research, official coroner's report, and agreements from all research partners involved, should have been submitted to the research committee for scrutiny. One wonders why members of these committees allowed themselves to be deceived by the applicants. Applications omitting vital information should have been rejected by those who are experienced in the approval process.

The case above emphasises the necessity and urgency that the working of the LRECs in each location, should be audited by an independently constituted panel, including lay people appointed to ensure objectivity. An appropriate training programme should be instituted prior to new members taking up their membership, with special attention being given to lay members. One also needs to raise the question of whether the individuals on these committees are suitably qualified.

Indeed, a number of initiatives within the EC and the UK, between 2004 and 2005, have now initiated reform of the research ethics approval system. Lord Warner has put forward a number of recommendations to reform the system in England, and is awaiting government response for its implementation.

There is also a question about the suitability of LRECs as the most appropriate committees to deal with research that involves clinical trials, and the use of organs and other human material. Dealing with research concerned with the development of medical products, the EU directive – 'the implementation of good clinical practice in the conduct of clinical trials on medicinal products for human use' – may also offer some guidance on good practice in other medical areas.[6] The purpose of the directive is to: (a) protect the rights, safety and well-being of the participants in research and (b) simplify and harmonise regulatory processes.

There can be no disagreement with the first aim, which is protecting the researched subjects. It is difficult to fully understand what may be meant by the second aim – simplification and harmonisation of regulatory processes could pave the way for further research that turns out to be ill-advised, due to greater 'simplicity'.

The Medical Research Council recently implemented the EU Directive (2001/20/EC)[6] stating that '[the] research organisation [is] to demonstrate promptly to MRC on request that the required permissions [i.e. regulatory authorisations and research ethics committee approval] are in place, or were in place when the activity occurred' (MRC, 2004).[7] The EU directive for clinical trials also requires research organisations/researchers responsible for the development of medicinal products or trials requiring human subjects to have a clinical trial authorisation and a sponsor. The sponsor is defined as 'an individual, company, institution or organisation which takes responsibility for the initiation, management and/or financing of a clinical trial' (MRC, 2004).[7]

To what extent these new initiatives will help to improve rigour in the research and ethics approval process remains to be seen. Introducing new policies and procedures is more easily attained than policing them. At present one would suggest that lay people would be fairly critical of the regulatory mechanisms for medical research, especially following the TGN1412 untested drug trial at Northwick Park hospital briefly mentioned in Chapter 1.

Increasingly the media is both more involved in, and successful at, enhancing public awareness of medicine and medical research. The *Guardian* recently reported the findings on the use of Herceptin outside clinical trials. The previously cited 10–26% of patients who experienced cardiac problems could be even higher. The US Food and Drug Administration warned that Herceptin could result in congestive heart failure or a dysfunction in the heart's ventricular chamber; their findings are further supported by the latest study which reported that one out of the 173 patients taking Herceptin in this study died from a cardiac related condition due to toxicity of the drug.[8]

This is not an isolated incidence regarding drug side effects. For example, in 2005, GPs were required by NICE (National Institute for Clinical Excellence) to stop prescribing anti-depressants for those under 18, as the drugs made them more likely to have suicidal thoughts.[9] How confident can one be about the research approval process? It is debatable whether these drug associated deaths could be regarded as clinically negligent issues. However, if these deaths could be shown to be the result of clinical negligence, then public trust in the medical profession would be further eroded.

Negligence

Negligence is a major cause of public distrust in a profession. There are a number of ways of defining negligence. Commonly, it could imply carelessness, inattentiveness and omission in attending to one's tasks, or abdication of responsibility. It could be seen as a failure to do one's duty, or a deliberate act to ignore one's obligations, or outright disobedience. It could be seen as a disrespectful act. It is a form of lawlessness that involves a determination to defy authority or to waive the rules.[10]

My own study on negligence came to the conclusion that negligence in professional practice can assume many forms, namely:

- lack of assiduity
- knowingly ignoring instructions given by the patient, his/her relatives and other professional associates

- actively and knowingly contravening laws of practice
- conscious acts resulting in physical injury or loss of dignity, individuality and autonomy of the patient and the relatives.[11]

These categories of negligence can be applied to many issues raised in previous chapters.

The accusation of lack of diligence can be applied to van Velzen as a medical practitioner in paediatric pathology, as he failed to carry out post-mortem examinations according to prescribed standards of practice. Many doctors at Alder Hey could be criticised for the lack of attention given to a specific law regulating autopsy practice. Ignorance of professional and legal regulations is a form of negligence.

One of the issues identified by the relatives was doctors' disregard of their personal instructions regarding post-mortem examination and the removal and retention of organs. Knowingly ignoring instructions constitutes a form of professional negligence. Members of the public provided evidence that their instructions to the pathologists were not heeded. There is evidence in the Chief Medical Officer's Summit report[12] and at public meetings that specific permissions for minimally invasive post-mortem examinations were given, but that these were ignored. Consent from parents and relatives for only small pieces of organs or tissues to be taken and retained, was flagrantly disregarded. The evidence would seem to suggest that the doctors had either misinterpreted the relatives' instructions or intentionally ignored them. Knowingly ignoring instructions given by the patients' relatives, either verbally or non-verbally, equates with the notion of hearing but not heard, seeing but not seen. The needs and requests of the families were not fulfilled, and the doctors had knowingly failed in their professional responsibility.

Instructions from parents and the families could be either implicit or explicit. During the consent process for a post-mortem examination, a parent or surviving relative might signal reservations, verbally or non-verbally, either because of religious belief, or as part of more general, but strongly-held ethical views. The doctor is professionally obliged to address such views. To ignore any doubts or any requests or instructions from patients or from families, and certainly to be selective about actual consent terms, must qualify as negligence.

The final category of professional negligence is concerned with any conscious acts that tend to dehumanise. From time to time, the public asks whether medicine has lost its humanity. What do people mean by that? Although we may accept that we are not altogether different from other animals, we would be indignant if told that our behaviour as human beings is fundamentally no different from theirs. We might argue that one of the major differences may be that human actions, although driven by desires,[13] can be distinguished from those of other creatures, by the fact that human beings have both the power to eliminate from choices presented to them, and to choose actions which are in accordance with laws. A hungry animal would prey upon other animals. A person possessing rationality – having the ability to reason – would abstain from such an action since it would be considered as cannibalistic by society. In the case of an animal, killing for food is a predatory response to hunger, whereas in the case of a person, the choice to kill is deliberate. This is one of the main characteristics of humanity. Kant, for example, defines humanity as 'the functional complex of abilities and characteristics that enable us to make rational choice.'[13]

In the context of organ retention, is it rational to deceive? Is it rational to undertake activities in medicine that will inherently diminish human values, provoke anger and disharmony? The medical profession is being challenged by these questions. We may need to dip into philosophy to answer the question of the meaning of loss of humanity in medicine. It means straying from the rational path. As is discussed in Chapter 1, some scientific activities are not rational.

Medical practice is within the confines of human action since it is concerned with the healing and curing of the sick; with helping individuals gain happiness and harmony in their world changed by illness and death; with effecting change in the patient's personal world through the practical application of the healing and curing art; with restoring health while, wherever possible, enabling the patient to maintain dignity and self-esteem; with effecting change in the world of suffering by bringing love and comfort to those who require it. The changes effected in the patient's personal world and in the world of suffering, are deliberate and performed in accordance with professional laws.

The achievement of such an aspiration by a practitioner in medicine would be an experience in the transcendental realm, which is, in Kantian and Husserlian terms (Edmund Husserl is a philosopher and founder of a European philosophy called phenomenology), attained by forgetting one's desire, self-interest or self-inclination and 'making the actions one takes become one's consciousness which reflect one's thinking, feelings and willing.'[14] The reflection of oneself requires a process of review within one's consciousness. This implies that whatever a doctor does is done as a human being, ensuring that actions are under his/her personal control. Therefore, actions which are brought about by the amalgamation of the body and the mind are not contaminated by desires, self-interest or anything that is less than 'good'. Therefore, 'doing good' becomes the sole preoccupation of the doctor.

It may be an ambitious leap from the practical problems of Alder Hey to such reflections. But the families did question doctors' humanity – 'Has medicine lost its art, ethics and humanity?'[15] A possible seat of problems in the NHS might consist in the failure to some extent of the humane standards of doctors. In the context of organ retention, one could argue that medicine as a profession has been putting its own interests, e.g. education, training and research, above the welfare of the patients and families. Much unhappiness has been caused to the families as the old wound of losing a child or a member of the family has been reopened. The world of the bereaved families has been turned upside down.

If one were to apply Kant's moral rules, it should be within the power of the doctor to enable the bereaved families to seek happiness and achieve harmony, rather than to compound grief. When the idea of happiness is translated into practice, it is concerned with things or actions intended to protect the living, to promote human values, to cure and to care for the sick, the infirm, the disabled, those who are vulnerable, the dying and the dead. Such actions are considered to have 'intrinsic worth'.[11] The following examples might suggest that organ retention is an act devoid of reason, therefore it is an irrational act, resulting in bodily mutilation of the dead and psychological injury to those who are having to deal with the consequences of such an irrational act. In many cases, this includes multiple funerals as outlined below.

Case 1: [They] were shocked to learn [their boy's] brain had been removed, kept for tests, then incinerated along with other parts, without their knowledge.[16]

Case 2: A mother whose 10-week-old son died of cot death syndrome [told] that doctors removed 25 organs and body parts, without her permission. 'There is something I would never ever let them take – like his tongue.' When [the mother] buried her son she was unaware that his heart, lungs, parts of his brain, and most of his tongue, had been taken away. She said: 'I have been visiting the grave every day for 14 years but now I am being told the hospital had more of my son than I have.' After organs had been returned, she said: 'We're going to bury [the little boy] all over again with his organs in a casket so he can finally be left in peace.'[17]

Case 3: Organs including hearts, lungs and brains were stripped from 88 cot death babies without the consent of their grieving parents. Parents are agonised over the scandal. They [organs] were kept in buckets, one marked 'unidentified trimmings.'[18]

Case 4: A [nine-month-old child] died 13 years ago from a virus, mother realised that the baby she buried was a shell. Most of the vital organs inside her tiny body were missing. [The mother] was told 13 years later that her daughter's organs were removed and retained during a post-mortem examination. 'She had had so many injections and needles inside her and when she died I felt she was finally at peace.' The mother said: 'We thought we had buried her with dignity. We thought we had dealt with it once. But now we haven't even got a chance to deal with it again [as the organs had been disposed of by the hospital]. The feeling I have is one of grief. And I also feel guilty that I did not bury her properly.'[19]

Case 5: 'When I was told, I was sick. I was physically sick, I never ever imagine[d] that the list of what they kept could have been that long. The hospital retained:

- all his brain, spleen, trachea, larynx, thymus, both lungs, both kidneys, tongue, mesentery, ileo-caecal valve with three vertebrae
- part of his heart, liver, rectum, stomach, testes
- tissue samples of his skin, bladder, spinal cord, pancreas, pituitary gland, and prostate gland.

'I am so angry. They stole my boy's soul. There was nothing left but an empty shell.'[20]

Case 6: 'I then buried around 100 pieces of my baby, kept in blocks and slides. They said they only kept pieces of millimetres thick but there were big chunks of his organs. It's like they did a pick and mix of his body, they butchered him. They did not use any of it for research.'[21]

The incidents cited above from newspapers represent only a very small number of families having the same experience throughout the United Kingdom. The incidents reported by newspapers can be corroborated, as similar accounts have been heard during the last three years at public meetings held by the Retained Organs Commission.

The theme of deceit has emerged as a major complaint against the doctors and the health service, and has been substantiated by various official reports. The families condemn the practice of deceit. According to Kant, being honest is the duty of a moral agent (a moral agent is defined as a person having the ability to think, judge and reason). This means every person in human society is a moral agent. Therefore any action emanating from this person is based on reason.

One of the most disturbing facts revealed by families affected by organ retention, is the feeling that their children and relatives had not been laid to rest because they had not been buried whole. The families feel guilty that their children and relatives had not been buried properly, and they felt that inappropriate respect had been afforded to the dead. The practice of routine 'stripping'[3] of a body's internal organs at post-mortem examination is regarded as undignified, disrespectful and irreverent. Parents and families object to the way in which specimens of body parts are kept – in buckets and jars and on shelves, and treated as disposable objects – to be incinerated. The Liverpool Children's Hospital reports that some specimens of eyes were not used for research (*see* Chapter 2). The families regard the practice of removing, retaining, storing and disposing of organs as dehumanising. Would any form of dehumanising action which diminishes self-esteem, reduces one's dignity and self-respect, both for the living and the dead, be regarded as a form of professional negligence?

One could argue that medical science lacks compassion in its approach to patient care. Compassion is defined by the Dalai Lama as 'a state of mind which is non-violent, non-harming and non-aggressive. It is a mental attitude based on the wish for others to be free of their suffering and is associated with a sense of commitment, responsibility and respect of others.'[22] No one would suggest that doctors and the medical profession would intentionally cause grief and unhappiness to those whom they intend to serve. This would be against all common sense. The counter-argument is: can human actions of any form be unintentional? If one re-examines many of the case studies in this work, there could be little doubt that the distrust of the public in the medical profession is well founded.

Regaining trust

During the course of the debate between 1999 and 2004, the medical profession has come to realise that the public has totally rejected the previous practice of post-mortem and of retention of organs. The public defies the medical authority. One consequence of this is that pathology, which is an important branch of scientific medicine, is under a cloud of mistrust. Pathologists have expressed strong concern that the Alder Hey disclosure has deterred doctors from undertaking pathology training. There are indications that members of the public will refuse consent to post-mortem examinations, and that people will cease to be willing to give their organs for teaching and research. As a result, the standard of medical practice could be seriously affected in the future.

Public awareness of the importance of pathology for healthcare should be stressed here. The public is also fully aware of the problems associated with previous standards of pathology practice. Since the public outcry, a number of serious deficiencies have been highlighted, including variations in standards of autopsy performance. The Royal College of Pathologists and the Department of Health for example, have recognised the need for new guidelines for autopsy practice. The College of Pathologists states: 'It is important that the autopsies that are undertaken now are performed to high standards, and that there is consensus amongst pathologists, their employers and the public over what those standards comprise. The comprehensive reviews of pathology practice extend also to the autopsy: there is need for review and a formal set of guidelines on autopsy practice.'[23]

The practice in the past should have been undertaken to the highest standard since one of the aims of autopsy is to enhance medical knowledge and to improve care. Now the public expects in the future that standards of practice will be uniformly applied and that serious deficiencies will be removed. Furthermore, the public expects that those who have responsibility for monitoring standards should exercise due diligence. The public further demands respectful and sensitive communication with bereaved families, enabling them to make important decisions at a difficult time. The public will have more confidence in the profession if there is evidence to show that lessons from the past have been learned, and a more stringent approach to monitoring behaviour of pathologists, and that rigorous standards of pathology practice are in place. Furthermore, the system must be open and transparent, allowing the public to participate in the inspection process where appropriate.

We are now familiar with the concept of 'institutionalised racism', the criticism directed at the Metropolitan Police force after the murder of Stephen Lawrence. Since then, other institutions such as the NHS and many large organisations have also been implicated. One could interpret institutional racism as a form of institutional negligence – either the alleged offence has occurred because those in charge of the organisation have been bypassed, or there is a deliberate policy to discriminate against certain groups of people, or to advance certain practices. One could argue strongly in the light of the Isaacs Report, that there has been discrimination against some members of the public, e.g. those who practise specific faiths, those who are incapacitated. The difficulty is to determine who will ultimately be responsible for the alleged offence. How will those involved be brought to justice, if there is a case to answer? The image of the institution could be irreparably damaged if justice is not seen to be done.

In addition to the negligence of individual doctors and groups of NHS managers within the spheres of post-mortem examination and organ retention, the healthcare institutions, including the government departments, the research organisations, the funding bodies, the gatekeepers of research ethics, could be said to be in breach of their collective responsibility by not upholding the law on the use of human tissue and body parts for teaching, education and research, and allowing the continuation of an inappropriate practice for many decades. The public questioned whether the principle of duty, i.e. 'care with due care' had been strictly followed by the whole system.

According to Kant, the notion of duty is one where action is not compelled by self-interest or other inclinations. An action done from duty has its own moral worth, not from the results it attains or seeks to attain, but from the principle of doing one's duty whatever that may be. The notion of duty is concerned with unconditional goodness, such as 'ought', 'right' and 'good'. These can be regarded as imperatives in professional practice, and should be upheld by all.

Who should be upholding these professional imperatives? The public would expect both individuals and the institution to apply the Kantian principle of duty to patients and all health service users. The public expects that the NHS institution would ensure that its practitioners, and other bodies carrying out its corporate functions, would follow government legislation. In August 1977 the Department of Health issued a circular in relation to the Human Tissue Act 1961, to instruct relevant personnel to follow a particular line of practice. The circular referred to was HC (77)28 entitled 'Removal of human tissue at post-mortem examination – Human Tissue Act 1961.' The first paragraph sets out its purpose: to facilitate 'the removal of organs and tissue, e.g. pituitary glands, during post-mortem examination for subsequent use for the treatment of other patients, and for medical education and research.' The same paragraph comments: 'It would be tragic if insufficient pituitary glands became available, since it is at present impossible to synthesise human growth hormones.'[4]

Institutional pragmatic interests can clearly dominate decisions at the corporate level, expressed as the will to achieve the public's good. The institutional pronouncement may be sadly at odds with the doctor's rational values, but the scientific desire to cure something untreatable may overcome *a priori* principles. The instruction issued by the Department of Health in August 1977, regarding the removal of pituitary glands without consent from the deceased's relatives, could be construed to be a covert institutional operation. Therefore it was unlawful, even if the intention was for the public's good. Did such a health policy inspire public confidence?

The matter of collective and institutional malpractice in medicine and the NHS is rarely discussed, as it opens up a range of difficult managerial, social and ethical issues. To do so could be to implicate many high-ranking officials in the health service, up to and including individuals in government. Can it be that finding individual culprits suits those responsible for the system all too well?

References

1 Department of Health. Good doctors, safer patients – proposals to strengthen the system to assure and improve the performance of doctors and to protect the safety of patients. A report by the Chief Medical Officer. London: Central Office of Information; 2006.

2 The Bristol Royal Infirmary Inquiry. The report of the public inquiry into children's heart surgery at the Bristol Royal Infirmary 1984–1995. London: The Stationery Office.

3 The Royal Liverpool Children's Inquiry. The Royal Liverpool Children's Inquiry report – summary and recommendations. London: The Stationery Office; 2001.

4 The Isaacs Inquiry. The Isaacs Report – the investigation of events that followed the death of Cyril Mark Isaacs. London: The Stationery Office; 2003.

5 The Shipman Inquiry. The Shipman Inquiry 3rd report – Death certification and the investigation of deaths by coroners. London: The Stationery Office; 2003.

6 The EU Directive for clinical trials. [Accessed 2005]. Available from http://www. ncrn.org.uk/portfolio/downloads/EU Directive.routemap.doc.

7 Medical Research Council/Department of Health. Joint Project in EU Clinical Trials Directive. www.mrc.ac.uk/index/current-research-clinical_research_governance/current-eu-clinical_trials_directive/current-joint-project.htm.

8 Hall S. Study finds greater heart damage risk from Herceptin than thought. The *Guardian* 2006 Aug 15; 6.

9 Boseley S. GPs to stop prescribing antidepressants blamed for suicidal feelings in under-18s. The *Guardian* 2005 Sept 28:3.

10 Lloyd S, editor. *The Penguin Roget's Thesaurus*. London: Penguin Books; 1984.

11 Cheung P. Phenomenology of nursing. [PhD thesis] Southampton: Univ. Southampton; 1992.

12 Department of Health. Chief Medical Officer's Summit – proceedings; 2001 January 11. Computer-aided transcription by Harry Counsell and Co. London: Department of Health.

13 Kant I. *Groundwork of the metaphysics of morals*. Paton HJ, tr. New York: Harper Torchbooks; 1948.

14 Husserl E. *Ideas – general introduction to pure phenomenology*. Boyce Gibson WR, tr. London: George Allen & Unwin; 1931.

15 The Retained Organs Commission. Minutes of the 15th meeting held in Cardiff.

16 Ramsay S. Time for answers on the 'organ stockpile'. *Manchester Evening News*: 2002 July 17; 1–2.

17 Smith R. The hospital gave back our dead son with 25 body parts missing. *Daily Mirror*: 2002 April 20; 10.

18 Coles J. Organs taken from 88 cot death babies. *Bristol Evening News* 2002 April 20; 9.

19 Health Correspondence. Body organ outrage – I thought my baby was finally at rest. *Nottingham Evening Post* 2001 May 18; 5–7.

20 Health Correspondence. Body organ outrage. *Nottingham Evening Post* : 2001 June 7; 6–7.

21 Tither H. What happened to my baby's heart? *Manchester Metro* Trafford ed: 2002 November 8; 2–3.

22 HH Dalai Lama. *The Art of Happiness*. London: Penguin Books, 1982.

23 The Royal College of Pathologists. Guidelines on autopsy practice. Report of a working group of the Royal College of Pathologists. London: The Royal College of Pathologists; 2002.

Chapter 10

Ethics and the practice of informed consent

Consent issues – gaps between theory and practice

Some questions and comments have been raised consistently in the last few years by members of the public who were dissatisfied with the consent process for requesting post-mortem examinations:

- who has the responsibility for informing parents about the issues of retaining human material – why didn't the doctors tell us truthfully?
- if we had been told a post-mortem was required we would have said no
- we didn't remember being asked – we remembered a form being given to us to sign and it was for a post-mortem
- we didn't remember any information given to us, as we were so upset about our son/daughter
- why were all the organs removed if the cause of death was known?

The tenor of the questions and comments is centred on two key issues regarding non-compliance with the Human Tissue Act 1961 and the contravention of the Coroners Act: the right to consent and how consent is sought by doctors both for hospital-based or coroner's post-mortem examinations. The previous chapters in this book have highlighted a real dichotomy between what is right in theory and what actually happened in practice. The gap between the two is significant, and has serious implications from the practice point of view; one could argue that the flawed process could affect the quality of care, as neither the doctor nor the patient could have considered all the alternatives available. There are no adequate explanations for this gap between theory and practice. The medical profession admitted that paternalism was the cause, as doctors wanted to spare families and parents any distressing details. But in the light of the official inquiries in the last few years, the medical profession cannot possibly continue to use paternalism as a meaningful argument. The Human Tissue Act 2004 now clearly specifies that consent is an imperative and any person who acts unlawfully, i.e. taking without consent, will be punished under this new Act.

How is consent defined, and how will the principles of seeking consent be put into practice in the future? What improvements are required in the consent process in the NHS to ensure that doctors are on the right side of the law? The penalty is high for practitioners found to act outside the law, as this will involve a 'summary conviction to a fine or imprisonment for not exceeding three years, or to a fine or to both.'[1] However, the law only applies to the deceased person and the way his/her body may be used after death. Currently, there is no legal imposition on the medical profession to obtain consent prior to routine investigations or treatment interventions, though it is usual for consent to be obtained from patients for many hospital procedures and treatments.

The correct use of nomenclature is important, so as to avoid confusion and serious misinterpretation. Currently, different terms such as 'consent', 'valid consent', 'informed consent', and 'more informed consent' are used by different groups of practitioners, government and other organisations. 'Informed consent' is used by the World Medical Association Declaration of Helsinki and the National Commission for the Protection of Human Subjects of Biomedical and Behavioral Research.[2] The Department of Health's guide to consent for examination or treatment[3] uses the term 'valid consent' to describe consent given voluntarily by a suitably informed person, who has the capacity to consent to an intervention. In practice, 'informed consent' and 'valid consent' are often used to mean roughly the same thing, i.e. consent is valid only if it is properly 'informed'.[3]

Since the organ retention malpractice has become public, most hospitals have redrafted their autopsy consent forms and refined the consent procedures to make them 'more informed'. What does 'more informed consent' mean? If the meanings of these terms are unclear, problems revealed in the past will recur.

The Independent Review Group on Retention of Organs at Post-mortem in Scotland preferred the term 'authorisation' (2001)[4]. 'Authorisation' is more meaningful from a common usage point of view. It leaves no room for misinterpretation. For example, if one says: 'I authorise you to sell this piece of furniture or a clock for me, at no less than a certain price,' then you may sell the object but not for less than the quoted value. However, the differences that exist within the English and Scottish jurisprudence systems could present difficulties for those practitioners who are able to work in the various countries of the UK. In principle, the existence of different definitions, in different countries, should not prevent someone from acting ethically and within the law.

The government has introduced the concept of 'appropriate consent.' 'Appropriate consent' in the Human Tissue Act 2004, as applied to adults, means personal consent if the person is still alive; or consent in writing if the person has died and the activity is one to which subsection 4 of the Act applies.[1] It is important to note that consent in writing must be one that was in force before the person's death.

Does this mean that the term 'appropriate consent' will have to be adopted by all whenever situations arise concerning the use of the human body? The prime rationale of obtaining consent is:

- the giving of information by the person seeking consent
- ensuring the information given is understood, and
- that consent is willingly, or voluntarily, given.

The legal system has a key role in determining the correct nomenclature, as it is worth noting that at present the term 'informed consent' is not recognised by English law.[3] This means that consent in this context is not legally imposed on the medical professional. This might mean that medical practitioners could withhold information from the patient if they believe this to be appropriate. Will the public be happy with this approach?

So far the subject of consent has not been a concern for legal compensation in England, as all the claims are concerned with clinical negligence.[5] However, after several landmark cases in the US, the issue of consent is now of broader social and political interest to the users of the health service and the medical profession. In one particular case – Natanson v Klein, the court ruled that the failure on the part of the doctor to provide adequate and appropriate information concerning treatment meant that the patient was not able to give informed consent. It was ruled as a case of negligence.[6]

In order for consent to be valid, the patient must have the minimum amount of information to understand both the object of the consent and the risks involved.[7] If that US ruling could be applied in the English courts, the 2900 cases of 'retention of organs and tissues following post-mortem examination' cited by the Department of Health[5] could be treated the same legally because taking the organs from the deceased would be deemed unlawful as the relatives have not been wholly informed of the purpose. The main difference between the Natanson v Klein situation and the organ retention affair is that the former deals with the living whereas the latter is concerned with the dead, particularly in relation to the issue of risks. The question of whether the cases of organ retention could be regarded as cases of negligence is a matter for scholars of medical jurisprudence. The important issue from the Natanson and Klein case is the quality of the consent process. This will be discussed later in this chapter.

At present, it is important for the medical profession and the health service to achieve uniformity in the way the concept of consent is put into practice, since the practice of consent is equally, if not more, relevant to living subjects. The Department of Health provides a set of general principles to be used when seeking consent for the removal and retention of human organs and tissue, and these could be used as the basis for further deliberations on how consent ('appropriate consent') might be translated into practice.

The general principles set out by the Department of Health are that:

- patients must be provided with suitable information in a form that they can understand. For example, they need to know that tissue of varying sizes may be removed as part of a surgical intervention, and that small pieces of tissue may be placed in blocks (of wax) or slides for examination under microscope, and possible retention
- they have the opportunity to ask questions
- they are able to give either explicit consent to particular tissue storage, or its use for teaching, research or therapeutic purposes
- they must give consent voluntarily without pressure or under undue influence
- in the case of children under 16 who are unable to give consent, parents or others close to the patient may be asked to give consent, though children with sufficient understanding of what is proposed may have the capacity to give effective consent
- where someone has died without giving an indication of his/her wishes as regards organ or tissue use, the responsibility for taking decisions, including whether a hospital post-mortem examination may take place, rests at present with relatives, or those closest, to the deceased person.[2]

In theory, the guidance set out above, though specifically prescribed for seeking consent for the removal and retention of human organs and tissues, could be applied generally to all situations in the NHS where consent is required for physical examinations, medical or surgical interventions, both minor and major.

It is interesting to note that, in practice, the guidance is not well observed. The patient's right to give consent to physical examination, particularly with regard to more intimate procedures, such as vaginal or rectal examinations, are often carried out by doctors without specific consent being sought. They are seen as part of the routine physical examination of hospital patients. The patient simply accepts that it was the duty of the doctor to conduct these physical examinations. Similarly, patients are rarely asked for consent before a venepuncture procedure (taking blood specimens for routine examination) is carried out. These routine procedures are taken for granted, as part of a doctor's duty in admitting patients to hospital. To what extent this current practice contravenes the code of professional conduct and the Human Rights Act, needs researching. The following example further demonstrates concerns relating to consent in respect of routine medical procedure, such as blood-letting for laboratory examination:

> A person from Africa fell ill during her visit to London. She was admitted to a hospital. She knew she was suffering from malaria. When in a hospital ward, two doctors decided to take a blood sample amounting to three test tubes of blood, because the doctors thought she was possibly HIV positive or else was suffering from AIDS. The husband enquired why that amount of blood was necessary for testing and he was told of the reason after the blood sample was taken. The husband believed that action taken by the doctors was uncalled for.
>
> (Author's personal notes, 2002)

The woman was not told why that amount of blood was necessary, but the patient was in no position to refuse as she might be thought to be a public health risk. The action taken by the doctors could be construed in the US as physical assault. If the patient was suspected to be HIV positive, that patient should have been informed of this by the doctor concerned and consent should have been sought for the said procedure to be carried out.

Some members of the public specifically complained about not having been told about the overall procedures of post-mortem examination. Others asserted that they did not understand the specific implications of what was asked of them. The process of seeking consent is not a mere formality, but demands that the person from whom consent is sought understands fully and accurately the 'procedure and risks and [needs] to respect the limits of their understanding, and of their capacities to deal with difficult information.'[8] In the case cited above, the doctor knowingly withheld information from the patient or gave wrong information during the process of seeking consent; this cannot be regarded as other than ethically impermissible. A reading of the Nuffield Council of Bioethics text would suggest that medical practitioners failed to do their ethical best to communicate accurately what was asked of members of the public. Thus, in spite of the signature on the consent form, however carefully obtained, the criterion that 'consent is fully informed'[8] was not met.

The quality of the consent process is influenced by several factors, namely:

- the types and quality of information, including any associated risks, given to the person concerned
- how the information is given and by whom

- the quality of the communication skills of the person seeking consent
- the circumstances in which consent is requested, i.e. the stress level of the person at the time
- the level of comprehension of the person from whom consent is sought.

The National Commission for the Protection of the Human Subjects of Biomedical and Behavioral Research recommends that information given to those who volunteer to take part in research[2] must include the purpose of the project and how it might benefit the population at large, the research procedures and their purpose, the risks involved, and alternative procedures which are normally applied if an innovative procedure is being tested. Verbal information must be accompanied by a written statement offering the opportunity to ask questions and to withdraw from the project.[1] Guarantees should also be given that withdrawal would not jeopardise the right to treatment or the relationship between the researcher and the subject. The risks associated with the project should be written in unambiguous language. If new drugs are used in clinical trials, subjects must receive written information on the risks associated with the untested drug in all circumstances, including any immediate reactions, and side effects in the longer term. Such detailed information will enable subjects to fully understand the implications in taking part in the project. These principles should be applied to every trial, however simple.

The serious reactions to TGN1412, the untested drug administered by Parexel in 2006, would suggest the importance of giving full information to research participants. The term 'cytokine release' was used in the consent form in the TGN1412 trial, which is totally incomprehensible to most lay people. In common language, the term means that the drug may make your body produce large quantities of inflammatory chemicals, called cytokines, which could cause headaches, shivering, back and gut pain, diarrhoea, swelling and nausea. How many of the six volunteers in the TGN1412 trial, would have been willing to take part if this had been explained? In addition, any findings from the animal phase testing should be revealed to potential participants at the consenting stage, to enable an informed decision. In some ways, the responsibility then lies with the individuals concerned, from the legal point of view.

The Department of Health states that 'consent is only valid if it is properly informed.'[3] This raises further questions of whether the information given, both verbal and written, has been fully understood by the person giving consent. What assessment is carried out to ascertain the level of understanding? What action would be taken in a situation where confusion occurs? These questions present some practical difficulties and challenges.

One of the prerequisites of ensuring 'valid consent', as defined by the Department of Health, is the qualification and experience of the health professional or the researcher who initiates the consent process, assuming the information being given is adequately prepared, as discussed previously. There have been many discussions in the last few years between the Retained Organs Commission, the public and doctors about who should seek consent from patients and relatives.

One needs to consider the customary arrangements in hospital where consent is obtained as a rule either by a nurse or a junior doctor. The consent form is given to an adult patient to sign, following some brief explanations about the operation and, usually without the presence of his/her relative. Little time is given to the patient to think about risks, or other implications, associated with the procedure for which consent is sought. In most cases, the patient would not expect to ask questions, as it is assumed that discussions have already taken place with the consultant or the medical registrar in charge of the procedure, and the procedure is then hurriedly carried out. Within the hospital establishment there is not a designated person in charge of the consent procedure, though there is a policy regarding consent.

A designated trained senior person in a hospital trust should be responsible for managing the process of consent. This person should oversee the policies and procedures applied in the health establishment. There should be trained staff in each ward who are qualified for this purpose and who need to be monitored and regularly updated. To avoid the possibility of anyone giving consent under duress, someone appointed by the patient, or by the deceased's relative, should be present when the consent is sought. If possible, i.e. where medical intervention is not considered life-threatening, there should be time allowed for the person from whom consent is sought, to discuss the matter with his/her representative without the presence of a staff member. The consent form must be signed by the person from whom the consent is sought, by the patient's representative, and the staff member concerned.

In practice, the goal of obtaining voluntary consent without duress is extremely difficult to achieve, as in most circumstances those from whom consent is required are highly stressed. Are there additional safeguards to ensure that the consent process is not hurried, and that patients and relatives have fully understood the procedures to which they are voluntarily giving consent? Are there lessons to be learned from other countries? The issue of consent is not a matter confined to the NHS in the UK.

A study carried out at Queen Victoria Hospital in Adelaide, Australia[9] concurs with the author's experience and observation, and with the experiences of members of the public in the UK. In the Adelaide studies, the researchers concerned knew of the dissatisfaction felt by the women from whom consent was obtained after perinatal loss. Care was taken to provide more detailed information at the consenting stage, and a counselling service was provided for bereavement support as part of the project.

A small group of 29 women took part in the above study,[9] of whom 19 had consented, and 10 refused consent, to a post-mortem examination of their dead baby. Both groups of women were asked about their satisfaction with the arrangements for post-mortem examinations after perinatal loss. This included women who had lost a baby through termination of pregnancy due to conditions diagnosed during pregnancy, to pregnancies that miscarried, to stillbirth or neonatal death. It is claimed that the women involved, prior to signing the post-mortem consent, were met by the doctors, and that they were counselled about the post-mortem procedure and the usefulness of the examination. Of those 19 who agreed to a post-mortem, at least 50% found the meeting with the doctors helpful, but said that neither the explanations about the procedure, nor the necropsy (autopsy), were useful. The other major criticism from those who were dissatisfied with the process was concerned with the clarity of the information presented to them during counselling. For example, one woman who had agreed to a necropsy (after counselling) assumed that the procedure was only tissue sampling.[9] The authors of the study concluded that a decision to consent to necropsy could not be regarded as an informed choice. One of the possible explanations in this case is that fear, anxiety and grief have been the main causes of non-comprehension amongst those consenting to post-mortem examination.[10]

A study examining parents' experience and views of post-mortem examination after losing their baby during pregnancy or infancy revealed that 'parents viewed the post-mortem examination as a useful tool in helping to discover the reasons why their baby had died.'[11] However, the doctors in this study recognised that there was a need to simplify the language used to explain findings enhancing 'parents' understanding of the value of post-mortem examination and ensure they are satisfied with it.'[11] The study further emphasised the importance of the medical staff being fully trained in the consent process, e.g. how to ask for parental consent, how to explain the post-mortem examination procedure and how to explain the findings.[11]

The capacity to deal with information, however simple, at a time when a person is most vulnerable (though no known research has been carried out to provide incontrovertible evidence of this), is almost certainly diminished as the person is suffering from physical and emotional stress. Nonetheless, this could be a contributory factor to the level of dissatisfaction expressed by the women in the studies in Australia and many parents involved in organ retention in the UK. In retrospect, those who had been in that situation and then recovered from the emotional shock, would possibly think that they might have been bullied into the situation.

The Bristol Royal Infirmary and the Royal Liverpool Children's Hospital Inquiries confirm that in some cases, doctors had on occasion exercised 'coercion' when families refused consent for a hospital post-mortem. When post-mortem examination requests in hospital were refused, deaths were referred to the coroner. Coercive actions are invariably wrong actions, since they 'fail to respect others or to accord them dignity, they injure human beings by treating them as things, as less than human, as objects for use.'[8] To presume consent fits with such a definition of coercion. Is it permissible for doctors to exercise presumed consent, even if the intention is to do good? The validity of presumed consent can be 'defeated by any one of numerous circumstances including violence, coercion, deception, manipulation, tendentious misrepresentation of the facts, and lack of disclosure of material facts or of conflicts of interests.'[8]

The Nuffield Council on Bioethics also criticised conduct that 'caused grave injury by treating one person's life or body or body parts as means to others' therapy or well-being without the relevant consent.'[8] Thus the staff of the paediatric cardiology centre in the Bristol Royal Infirmary inquiry were implicated in ethically questionable behaviour of organ retention as well as injury to the children. In the light of the Rahman/Khong and Rankin/Wright/Lind studies,[9,11] one should attempt to explore the issue of coercion objectively, and seek explanations for the behaviour of those doctors in Bristol, who are essentially caring. It might be that the information given by the doctors, particularly in verbal form, was not at all understood by parents, and that the parents were asked to make a decision too quickly.

Perhaps focusing on the part played by coercion in organ retention may strike the reader as a distraction. It is only a word. But let us stop to consider how most of us have personal experience of dealing with 'arm-twisting' requests and how difficult it is to say no for fear of upsetting others. For example, one might be approached by a superior to take on something extra at work. The request might be put in such a way that one has no alternative but to accept. The boss might say: 'It could benefit a lot of people if we were able to do such and such, but we haven't been able to find anyone to do these things yet. Since you have the experience and expertise, while realising extra pressure might be put on you, would you or could you seriously consider taking on these extra tasks until such a time as we are able to find someone else to do so? It would be good for your CV and future job prospects.'

The moral pressure (or blackmail) is on, and the person concerned is coerced into making a decision. Clearly, according to Nuffield's definition, coercion can range from what seems relatively mundane and harmless, to examples that involve deception and violation of an individual's rights. So the area for decision-making depends on how far such a definition is appropriate. Nuffield may define coercion so broadly as to place a question mark against any future proposal for an opt-out provision in respect of consent for use of organs. In other words, future regulation – likely to apply, perhaps, only to the present system of donor cards – that sought to assume consent to donation of organs in the absence of a registered withholding of consent, would be of doubtful ethical standing.

In the light of the published studies and inquiry reports, one cannot be totally convinced that any new system will improve the validity of the consent given, without changing the timing at which consent is sought. Even if bereavement counselling services are in place, and people are given the emotional support required both before and after the consent is signed, and even with improved doctor communication skills, some people will remain baffled at the end of the process. For consent to be valid, the Department of Health states that the information given must be 'properly understood', and that consent must be given voluntarily by a 'suitably informed person' or a 'reasonable person', who has the capacity to consent to intervention (intervention applies to treatment for a living person). To what extent can a person be described as 'reasonable' when emotionally confused and numbed? Assuming that someone is in a state of shock and confusion, cannot fully understand complex details, then the consent obtained in this state cannot be regarded as valid. Even if someone is, or appears to be, in a fit state to make important decisions in spite of the emotional stress, can the consent given be said to be given voluntarily? The consent obtained under these circumstances could be argued as invalid, since it is obtained under emotional duress.

Consent is necessary for the preservation of a person's right to self-determination; it is not something that is imposed by doctors. Health professionals may not see this as an appropriate attitude, as consent, perceived in this way, will impose restrictions on clinical practice. The latest clinical policy from the Nursing and Midwifery Council was that it would be permissible to hide 'patients' medication in food and drink, if it is deemed to be in their best interests.'[12] If the policy is implemented, then there is a licence for any medication to be given to confused or mentally incapacitated patients without their knowledge, because without it, their condition will deteriorate – a typical argument for something that is done in the patient's best interests. But is this ethical? The notion of something that is done in one's best interests, without one's consent, violates one's rights.

The paternalistic culture appears to be endemic within the health service. A recent study showed that nurses 'would badger patients into agreeing to procedures even when they initially refused consent.'[13] Another study found that nurses ignored the refusal of treatment from some patients because they believed the procedure was in the patients' best interest. One nurse admitted that she gave painkillers in syrup to a patient after the woman had refused drugs, as the nurse thought it was ludicrous to see the patient suffering.[13] Who is ultimately accountable for one's well-being? Is it the doctor or the nurse? Or is it the person himself or herself?

The statement, 'it is in the public's best interests or the patient's best interests', often comes from doctors, researchers, lawyers, government ministers. The term does not sit too comfortably with us, the members of the public and those who are concerned for our welfare and act on our behalf, since we are all part of society. The term is divisive as it creates a 'them and us' situation. You are a patient and you are to be treated. One feels belittled. Equally, one often hears the term, 'the ordinary people' or the 'ordinary people in the street.' What do these terms mean? One would suggest that every one of us is an ordinary person if we discard our professional identity. Even the prime minister or a president of a country can be an ordinary person. 'Ordinary person' seems derogatory as a term, as it implies that there is no significance attached to our presence in time and space. Being an 'ordinary person' means that one has no authority in a given circumstance and that one's autonomy is obfuscated.

It might be that this term is being used too loosely, and too frequently, within the public sector, where the assumed authority to act on behalf of others in society is taken for granted. Are we asked, for example, as members of the public, whether it would be appropriate to use brains obtained from deceased persons without consent, in order to conduct research? Medical researchers assume that no objections will be raised by the public, as it is believed the results of the research will be of benefit to some. The progress of such a research programme remains obscure, as it is believed that ordinary people would not want to know any more about it. On the contrary, many of us do want to find out what scientists are doing. Ordinary people do object from time to time to scientific experiments. It is not just a question of whether one is inside or outside the circle; it is simply easier to exclude those seen as outside the circle, i.e. the 'ordinary person' in the street and the patient in the hospital.

Improving the validity of consent

How will the validity of consent be improved in the future for those who will be asked to give consent on behalf of the deceased for whatever reason, and for those who require medical or surgical treatment?

Obtaining voluntary, informed consent from the patient for medical and surgical interventions is a practice that deserves the greatest care. It should be undertaken seriously by senior doctors, or at least by someone who is well qualified in this aspect of clinical work, even though it might not be seen as part of the clinical activity. The person responsible must be a permanent member of staff, which will exclude anyone who is not yet at medical registrar level. In addition, the designated doctor in charge of consent for a particular patient should have received sufficient training. There must be agreed mechanisms for inspection of the consent process on a regular basis, and lay people must be involved. It is recognised that the proposed change cannot be effected immediately, but there need not be undue delay. If delays are experienced, the future progress of medicine might well be jeopardised.

Consent for the removal and retention of organs would require a different process from that used in day-to-day clinical practice. The studies instigated by the Retained Organs Commission point out that, although there are those who are willing to give consent for their own post-mortem examination, they are more reluctant to make decisions on behalf of their relatives.[14] This further suggests that the current system of seeking consent needs a new direction.

The principal question one needs to address is: how will the validity of consent be improved in the future? One could nibble at the edges by making the information about post-mortem procedure more easily understood; by involving senior doctors and some pathologists when consent is sought, as suggested by many families; by employing counsellors and 'tissue nurses', whose focus is to enable the family to make an informed choice. These proposed improvements might be considered sound initially, but they still do not remove the fundamental problem, that of the deceased's relatives having to make an important decision about someone else's body at a most vulnerable time.

One possible alternative might be that a designated hospital official visits the family at home a few days after someone dies. The home environment will provide a more congenial setting in which difficult discussions can take place, in the comfort of one's home. Discussions at home will avoid any embarrassment caused when one is upset, particularly in the presence of other strangers in a hospital corridor. The chapel of rest in a hospital could be used for this post-mortem examination interview, where the chaplain and other relatives could be present to give support if necessary. In addition, the family should not be required to make, or be coerced into making, an immediate decision, even though the hospital authority might wish it. Additional time should be given to digest the information given and to examine the implications of refusing consent for post-mortem. This will offer the family a period to grieve privately and time to make an informed choice. The proposal is worthy of testing.

A more radical approach might be to move away from the accustomed practice. Instead of asking a deceased's spouse for consent to post-mortem examination, healthy individuals, partners, families, nominated persons, should be encouraged to think about post-mortem examination and the need for body organs for education and research and asked to made a decision before death. The proposed new approach will not only remove the undesirable psychological burden on the spouse imposed by the current system, it will also allow citizens to make a genuine and informed choice for themselves, similar to making a will in advance. The suggested approach is similar to that used for blood donor and organ donor recruitment; it will enhance the validity of the consent given, as it will negate the problem of making a decision for someone else.

The current rules regarding children under 16 years of age and those who are not competent to make a decision, will continue to apply (parents or guardians will be responsible for the child until the person reaches the consenting age of 16). One could even extend the approach to the prospective population; that is, parents are asked to make an advance directive, regarding post-mortem examination and donation of organs for education and research, as soon as a newborn arrives.

The successful implementation of such a reform takes time. It will also depend on:

- a shift in the existing attitude in society, and in the minds of the health professionals
- a change in social policy emanating from government departments
- a long-term education programme involving existing agencies responsible for blood transfusion, organ donation and transplantation services.

Since the policy change affects the public at large, it would seem sensible that the public should be widely consulted to establish whether there are any objections to such a proposal, and to seek suggestions on how best such a policy change might be achieved. It is important that opinion from a representative sample of all age groups should be sought, including schoolchildren. Schools should be encouraged to take an active part in the survey exercise. Since the public is unhappy about the previous practice, the findings of the public consultation exercise must be well publicised in unambiguous language.

For consent to serve a purpose, it must be specific. Members of the public told us in meetings that their consent for limited post-mortem examination seemed to have been used as authority for the doctors to examine other organs during post-mortem examinations. They had not given permission to remove or retain organs that were later unaccounted for. Legally, one would have thought intentionally ignoring consent given would constitute professional misconduct (see discussion elsewhere). For the future it may be noted that such action also apparently contravenes Article 11 of the Council of Europe draft Bioethics Convention.

The following accounts given by members of the public appear to suggest that terms of consent had been violated:

> '... I've found it difficult to forgive the deception and felt that body parts had been stolen after she had given what she believed was permission only for slivers of tissue to be taken at post-mortem. It made it worse that these body parts had never been used. Many [of us] would never again trust the hospital authorities...'[15]

> '... Many parents have offered organs for research and transplant. There had been deliberate deception, not simply done to spare parents' feelings. Parents had in many instances found that consent they had given had been ignored or violated...They [doctors] took my son's brain, his spleen, his testes, etc – what for?'[16]

> '... I gave permission to the doctors to remove the heart, but why were my son's other organs removed at the same time...'

The last question was typical of those repeatedly asked at Retained Organ Commission meetings.[17]

References

1 Human Tissue Act 2004: Elizabeth II. Chapter 30. London: The Stationery Office, 2004.
2 The National Institute of Health. National Commission for the Protection of Human Subjects in Biomedical and Behavioral Research. US: Maryland; 1979.
3 Department of Health. Human bodies, human choices – the law on human organs and tissue in England and Wales. A consultation report. London: Department of Health Publications; 2003.
4 Scottish Executive Health Department. Independent Review Group on retention of organs at post-mortem. Report on Phase 3. Edinburgh: Scottish Executive; 2003.
5 Department of Health. Making amends – a consultation paper setting out proposal for reforming the approach to clinical negligence in the NHS. A report by the Chief Medical Officer. London: Department of Health Publications; 2003.
6 Katz J. ed. Natanson v. Klein. *Experimentation with human beings.* New York: Russell Sage; 1972.
7 Kaufmann CL. Informed consent and patient decision making: two decades of research. *Soc. Sci. Med.* 1983; **17(21):** 1657–64.
8 Nuffield Council of Bioethics. Human tissue – ethical and legal issues. London: Nuffield Council on Bioethics; 1995.
9 Rahman AH, Khong TY, Survey of women's reactions to perinatal necropsy. *BMJ.* 1995; **310:** 870–1.
10 Knapp RJ, Peppers LG. Doctor-patient relationships in fetal/infant death encounters. J *Med Educ.* 1979; **54:** 775-80.
11 Rankin J, Wright C, Lind T. Cross sectional survey of parents' experience and views of the post-mortem examination. *BMJ.* 2002; **324:** 816-8.
12 Duffin C. Covert administration of drugs to be condemned. *Nursing Standard* 2003; **17(34):** 9.
13 Harrison S. Patients being badgered for consent to treatment. *Nursing Standard* 2004; **18(29);** 9.
14 Irvine Associate. Qualitative research to explore public perceptions regarding retention of organs and tissue for medical practice, teaching and research. Commissioned by the NHS Retained Organs Commission. London. 2002.
15 Retained Organs Commission. Minutes of the 6th meeting 2002 Oxford. London: The Retained Organs Commission.
16 Retained Organs Commission. Minutes of the 10th meeting 2002 Cambridge. London: The Retained Organs Commission.
17 Retained Organs Commission. Minutes of meetings between 2001–2004. London: The Retained Organs Commission.

Chapter 11

The medical profession and the public

Medical paternalism

From time to time the medical profession is challenged by serious incidents and has to re-examine its professional function and its relationship with the public. These challenges might seem unwelcome, but they provide an opportunity for the profession to ask some fundamental questions, such as: what is the basic professional philosophy of the medical profession; how must its members behave in all circumstances; how is the profession perceived by the public and what improvements are necessary to uphold practice standards and professional ethics? Some philosophers would suggest that the asking of these basic questions serves to reaffirm the meaning and purpose of the profession. Members of the public are users of the medical profession and the services are paid for by taxes. Doctors are public servants and, therefore, their purpose is to satisfy the health needs of those who are sick and vulnerable, and to provide protection to those who are healthy.

Much of the social interaction in hospital between the doctor and the public is in the consulting situation where the doctor makes the diagnosis and prescribes treatment. A member of the public, once in the consulting room, becomes a passive participant in the consultation process. Thus, the accustomed doctor and patient relationship is created. The ill person, once in the hospital consulting room will be asked to undress, to be examined and at the end of the consulting process, a case file will be produced. The doctor uses jargon to address the patient, and this language is seldom understood by the patient. The doctor, because of his knowledge and skills in medicine, carries authority and therefore assumes a superior stance in the consultation process. The patient normally listens to the verdict given, which sometimes appears cold and impersonal. The impersonal style of communicating diagnosis, or giving bad news to the patient or interacting with the patient, is meant to be kind and to avoid causing further distress. Such an entrenched attitude has been recognised by some members of the medical profession and described as 'cultural malaise'.[1] Some members of the public, especially those who have suffered serious harm due to clinical negligence, would say that this assessment is correct.

The expression 'doctor knows best' or 'you shouldn't go too close to a patient', might have originated from the traditional interaction described above, and has been criticised by some as the 'medical model of care', or the 'medical habit of mind'.[2] The medical habit of mind is associated with the method of doing things, with how doctors see things, with the basic concept of knowledge and science, with moral responsibilities, with the image of man. Generally, the body is seen as a thing, an object, for observation and technological manipulation.[2] More generally, the habits of mind adopted by doctors replicate their attitudes towards everyday life, specialised attitudes developed through an extension of professional practice, through teaching and research.

Each discipline within medicine is concerned with the development of knowledge in its own branch and advancement through research and perfecting of treatment. Research requires raw material, and the raw material has to be obtained from somewhere. For pathology, the main source of material is both the living and the dead. This discipline is partly concerned with the development of scientific techniques and diagnostic competence, i.e. how to preserve organs and fix tissues, etc; and how to develop diagnosis through careful examination of the object under the microscope, and it is carried out in the interests of the public and public health. This might be the way in which the medical profession is perceived by a lay person.

The medical habit of mind is deeply ingrained within the culture of medicine, and 'may be learned as a result of instruction or socialisation or may be picked up as one grows accustomed to certain ways and means of doing things.'[3] The public is suggesting perhaps that the accustomed habit of mind adopted by doctors through many generations be replaced by a more enlightened attitude, such as 'the patient first', and *primum non nocere* – first do no harm'. Such an attitude would require the medical profession to look at health and illness from a human point of view rather than an organic and mechanical one. Ian Kennedy, chair of the Royal Liverpool Children's Hospital Inquiry, indicates that there is a cultural problem within the medical profession. The accustomed habit of mind is difficult for colleagues and junior doctors to expose, as they are often threatened by victimisation.

In practice, the medical habit of mind has a tendency to remove a person's individual identity and right to make informed choices. The doctor tends to consider a person who requires treatment as his/her patient; one who has no right to accept, or object, to treatment or procedures prescribed. The patient is a passive object to be observed, diagnosed and treated. The patient is automatically deprived of the right to ask questions, to challenge practice. From the doctor's point of view, the treatment proffered is carried out in the patient's best interest. The following example shows the position of a person being a patient, under the accustomed medical model of care:

> A young research student was required to seek medical advice from his local hospital. He had been complaining of pain and being generally unwell. He knew the possibility that he might have contracted some tropical diseases in Africa as he had been conducting some research fieldwork in Africa for a few months. He had been under investigation but the condition worsened. He was admitted to the hospital for further investigations. A number of investigative procedures were prescribed including some internal x-ray procedures. However, nothing abnormal was detected from these investigations. Eventually he was told that some special blood samples would be required to be taken from the bone marrow of his hip bone (the procedure is considered invasive and painful as a sharp metal instrument relatively large in diameter will have to puncture the skin introduced through the bone prior to blood samples being obtained). No consent was asked for and the procedure went ahead. The student had no choice but to accept the treatment. He was found to be normal and additional treatment was prescribed after this traumatic procedure. The student remained unwell for some time.
>
> (Notes recorded by the author)

Does medical paternalism have a place?

Although the case above is partly concerned with the issue of consent discussed in a previous chapter, it is principally a manifestation of the accustomed culture within the medical profession; one which has never been challenged successfully by the public. The medical model of care reinforces the assumption of professional autonomy on the part of the doctors with a corresponding attitude of benign paternalism. Furthermore, the accustomed model of care provides the medical profession with therapeutic privileges, including withholding information or deciding a course of action without fully consulting the patient. However, that does not mean that the medical profession is right in the way it perceives its role. The above situation is not an isolated incident; this is how it operates throughout the NHS. It may be perceived by the medical profession that if the medical model of care were to be replaced by a partnership approach, where the patient's autonomy becomes more dominant, it will threaten the perceived legitimacy of the profession over patient's self-determination.

The term 'the medical habit of mind' is recognised by the medical profession, but phrased as medical paternalism, i.e. we don't want to distress the patient and his family further by being honest with them about the diagnosis and prognosis. Since the organ retention affair, it is now recognised by some as an undesirable and arrogant attitude. The then president of the Royal College of Pathologists apologised for the 'tremendous distress that parents and other relatives [had] suffered over this matter of organs and tissues retained following post-mortem examination of their loved ones.'[4]

As the representative of the college, he would reserve judgement about the outcome of the Alder Hey inquiry. He emphasised that 'they [doctors involved] were always acting in the interest of the families concerned and were trying to discover more about the precise cause of death and to learn about the diseases involved.'[4] He said further: 'The details of what were involved were seldom explained to the recently bereaved, [neither was there an intention] to deceive, [nor was it] because of arrogance or indifference, but plainly and simply to avoid further distress. That was in the past and we now fully realise and completely accept that this somewhat paternalistic approach may have been acceptable practice some years ago but is certainly not now.'[4]

One should really question the appropriateness of medical paternalism in the past, and, in particular, for the future. Can paternalism continue to have a place in the health service? Does the paternalistic culture serve to protect those for whom the service is provided? The rationale for this attitude might be that doctors need to be detached from human suffering, and to address the issues surrounding life and death from the clinical and scientific standpoint. It has also been argued that paternalism serves to safeguard clinical decision-making for the benefit of the patients, since a real problem of contemporary medical practice is that patients are bombarded with too much information. Patients may even feel sometimes that the burden of making clinical decisions is transferred to them.[5] It may be argued that if openness were to exist within the health service, it would only cause further damage. Doctors could be seen by patients as evading clinical responsibility.

Paternalism in the medical profession stems from genuine concern for the patient. It also serves to protect those who are vulnerable, for example, those who are not considered 'mentally competent'. What about the law itself with its paternalistic role of serving to protect by maintaining order? Paternalism can be seen as one expression of love inside a family, but the relationship between parents and child cannot inform the nature of a good doctor-patient relationship, which is a clinical one. A paternalistic model in medicine is positive in so far as it concerns what is best for the patient from the patient's point of view. However, this is contradicted by the evident reality that the patient usually wants to be fully informed of the situation so that he/she can make an informed choice. It is doubtful whether many doctors now believe that patients want their doctor to make the decision for them. However, issues of organ retention and consent around the time of death may have seemed, within the NHS of past years, to be a situation where paternalism was appropriate.

Surely today, while there may be some patients who would prefer their doctor to be in charge of the decision-making process, the patient must be kept fully informed of the reasons for the treatment decisions. Even if the patient decides that he does not want to know, the doctor must make sure that the patients fully understand the implications of the treatment offered. Paternalism would seem inappropriate in any given clinical situation.

Paternalism is defined by Wasserstrom as follows: 'By paternalism I shall understand roughly the interference with a person's liberty of action justified by reasons referring exclusively to the welfare, good, happiness, needs, interests, or values of the person being coerced.'[6]

Paternalistic action imposes restrictions upon individual freedom to act in one's own good, even if there has been no coercion. Is this true in every case? For example, in the case of a mentally incompetent person who is in danger of self-harm, a decision taken by a doctor could be permissible, so long as the next-of-kin or guardian is fully involved in the process. In this case, the issue of coercion does not apply. A problem might arise where the next-of-kin or the guardian of a mentally incompetent person cannot be contacted in time. Then, if a decision has to be taken to prevent serious injury to the person concerned, it can be taken for the person's own good, even though that person's liberty has been interfered with. Indeed, if the decision were not taken on this person's behalf, the doctors could be close to an accusation of professional negligence.

Although it has been suggested that a paternalistic attitude has no place in the future NHS, from an ethical point of view the central question of paternalistic medicine is whether paternalist action violates moral or natural laws or the code of conduct prescribed for the profession.

It might be helpful to use a hypothetical example to develop the argument as follows. Of two un-identical twin brothers, one suffers from chronic kidney failure and has been on maintenance haemodialysis (on a kidney machine) for some time. His condition has been deteriorating. He would only survive if he were to be given a kidney transplant. The patient agrees. However, the doctors experience considerable difficulty in obtaining a suitable donor kidney because of the patient's rare blood group, and the patient is deteriorating rapidly. The medical consultant and the surgeon seek permission, and obtain full consent, from the other twin for his kidney to be used in order to save the patient's life. (The hypothetical example might seem unlikely but doctors could be faced with this dilemma). However, the patient was not told of the origin of the donor kidney. Neither was the twin told of the associated risks both to himself and his brother. Should the patient have been told of the origin of the donor kidney?

The doctors could be said to have acted paternalistically towards the patient, as they believed the patient would benefit clinically from the kidney transplantation, and that there were minimal risks for both the patient and the donor. The risks of not performing the transplantation would put the patient at far greater risk. The doctors believed they were qualified to make clinical decisions on behalf of the patient, and the decision was taken entirely for the patient's own good. In the view of doctors, the patient, if consulted, would be able ethically to consent to his brother's gift. However, he might be unwilling to accept any risk for his brother, and be less than impartial – he might put his twin first. One might agree that the doctors' action was good, but according to Wasserstrom, the patient's liberty to choose had been infringed. In other words, acting without getting full consent is a form of deception, even without intention to deceive. No such rationale, as in that hypothetical case, applies in our context. Altruistic motives of families, arising from the memory of the dead child or adult relation, and invoked as part of the rationale, are surely a step too far in presuming consent. Doing good should not be imposed upon individuals.

Does the doctor in fact know best? Do the public want the doctor to make decisions for them? There are indications in this book that the public not only do not want the doctors to take charge of the decision, but in fact, they resent such protective attitudes and behaviour. The public want to participate in the process of making an informed decision for themselves. They want the doctor to advise them of the requirements at various stages of the illness journey. It is the personal decision of the patient to either accept, or reject, the treatment recommended by the doctor. Occasionally patients might refuse the treatment offered. For instance, a person who is diagnosed as suffering from depression might refuse prescribed anti-depressants, as in his/her experience, the side effects outweigh the benefits. In which case, the patient does know best.

If medical paternalism could be taken to mean a caring attitude, it should be cultivated rather than discouraged. Instead of saying 'I don't think the patient or his family should know the diagnosis,' the doctor should exercise his/her communication skills to find out how best the meaning of the diagnosis and treatment could be conveyed, without causing unnecessary distress. Inevitably it will be distressing to anyone with a diagnosis of a serious or terminal illness. The public expect honesty in all circumstances. Evading the issue of passing on distressing news might seem a good idea at the time, but in the end, the truth will have to be told.

All of us recognise that imparting unpleasant or bad news is an unenviable task for anyone. Having to explain procedures at a time of grief is clearly a tough job. Ideally, doctors and nurses should be trained in this important aspect of medical and nursing care. A close look at these and other case histories suggests that the fundamental complaint is of lack of openness in talking about post-mortem procedures. Trying to spare patients' feelings in a paternalistic approach may not be the only explanation, however. It is likely that inadequate training had not provided staff with any insight into their lack of knowledge and skills in communicating with the public.

The public expects sympathy and empathy from the doctor. Empathy is one of the most difficult attributes to demonstrate in a doctor-patient relationship.

It is a two-way process that implies a two-way participation between two human individuals, or the willingness of the individuals concerned to enter into reciprocal engagement, such as talking with each other, attempting to understand each other's moods and emotions and each other's feelings about things. Disengagement from this process can result in a one-sided affair and in communication failures. From the doctor's perspective, he has failed in his clinical responsibility, and from the patient's point of view, he has been let down.

Medical paternalism is perceived, from the public point of view, as a failure of the medical profession to listen, to understand and to change entrenched inappropriate attitudes. The criticism levelled at the medical profession by the public is real and the ethos of medical paternalism needs critical examination by practitioners themselves, and the profession as a whole.

In March 2004 there was a debate in a strategic health authority in which the author was involved. A medical member of the authority perceived as hysteria the grief and emotions displayed in the last few years by those members of the public involved in the illegal practice of organ retention. It was seen as an excessive reaction, resulting in a needless amount of financial resources being expended inappropriately, and causing a further decline in organ donation. The absence of a dissenting view from other members of the strategic health authority denotes that the view was shared by all. Such an erroneous perception of a practice, identified as an illegal one, does not inspire confidence that the ethos will change. Unless there is a real willingness to change within the profession, the relationship between the public and the profession will not improve.

The public does not seek to judge the professional behaviour of doctors, nor does it wish to be confrontational. The users of the health service seek to remind the profession how it ought to behave in all circumstances. In some ways, 'they [seek] to guide, not to instruct, but merely to show and to describe what I [they] see. All I [they] claim is the right to speak according to my [their] best lights...'[7]

References

1 Irvine D, Doctors in the UK: their new professionalism and its regulatory framework. *Lancet.* 2001; **358**: 1807–10.

2 Kestenbaum V, editor. *The Humanity of the Ill – phenomenological perspectives.* Knoxville: The Univ. of Tennessee Press; 1983.

3 Bensman J, Lilienfeld R. *Craft and consciousness: occupational technique and the development of world images.* New York: Wiley; 1973.

4 Department of Health. The Chief Medical Officer's Summit – proceedings. Computer-aided transcription by Harry Counsell and Co. London: Department of Health; 2001 January 11 2001:15.

5 Fitzpatrick M. Amnesty for dead organs: morbid anatomy. http://www.spiked-online.co.uk.

6 Wasserstrom R, editor. *Morality and the law.* Belmont CA; Wadsworth; 1970.

7 Husserl E. *Die Krisis der europäischen Wissenschaften und die transzendentale Phänomenologie.* Husserliana VI, 17. The Hague: Martinus Nijhoff; 1936.

Chapter 12

Empowering the public

The contribution of the voluntary patient groups

We must not underestimate the contribution of individuals and voluntary patient groups in bringing pressure to bear on the health service and the health professions to see the users' point of view and to bring about policy change. The personal price is high for individuals and members of the voluntary groups who became active in the pursuit of justice, equality of treatment, and a better service for others, as can be seen in the cases of Sally Clark and the families in Bristol and Liverpool. One would expect the care provided by the health service, social services and the legal service, to be of the highest standard, and users should not need to expend energy and resources in making their voices heard. The reality is different. It is important to examine the reasons for, and the basis upon which, patient voluntary groups or self-help groups are formed.

Patient voluntary groups, such as the National Childbirth Trust (NCT) and Scottish Care and Information on Miscarriage (SCIM) arose from some women's unhappy experiences of giving birth and nursing their children, and from unsympathetic attitudes of doctors and nurses in providing antepartum and postpartum care. SCIM was set up initially by a few socially committed women who were horrified by the impersonal and sometimes callous attitudes of nurses and doctors towards them, following a miscarriage. Members of SCIM felt that off-the-cuff unprofessional remarks, such as 'never mind, you can always try again', 'it doesn't matter as you have another nine to look after', proffered by health professionals about their misfortune, were humiliating. These were not the professional responses women either wanted, or expected, to hear from health professionals.

Those who founded SCIM were also concerned about the inadequacy of the immediate care given following a miscarriage, and the gross lack of evidence-based advice on planning for future pregnancies. Furthermore, members of SCIM believed that, not only did the clinicians fail to understand the clinical problems associated with threatened abortion, but, more importantly, they failed to understand the emotional plight of these women. Women felt their self-worth was grossly undermined as a result of not being able to carry their baby to full term, and the situation was made worse by the lack of sympathy and understanding shown by clinicians. SCIM was, therefore, set up as a drop-in centre for women to share experiences, to console each other in their grief and to find ways of helping each other to plan for the future.

The activities of groups such as SCIM have resulted in the production of a new policy by the Scottish Department of Health, on the management of early pregnancy loss.[1] Many similar patient groups have been founded by users of the health service out of a sense of desperation, as they felt the health service had failed them. The formation of these self-help groups was regarded as a positive action. In such situations, the helplessness and sense of desperation may bring about despondency and bitterness, which would have a negative impact on physical and emotional well-being, as seen in some families affected by the organ retention scandals. For example, the members of the Retained Organs Commission (ROC) were told by some parents in Liverpool, and elsewhere, that they were still, years later, finding it difficult to talk about their past experiences. Consequently these parents have been suffering unresolved grief in silence, and without any official support. A number of families said they had developed a sense of guilt: at one public meeting, some members of the public were brave enough to say: 'I wished I were strong enough to say no to the post-mortem'; 'Had I raised objections at the time, I would have buried my child whole'; 'I wish I had never left him at Alder Hey and I blamed myself for that'. A small number of parents have become unemployed due to mental ill health. However, out of these traumatic and unfortunate experiences, people have turned grief into something positive, as demonstrated by their resolve to help others through the many successful and well-run self-help groups. Most of these groups are self-financing, offering help, counselling and advice to those who have been through the same experiences.

Once the problem came to light of organ removal and retention without knowledge and permission of parents and relatives, many new support groups throughout England were established. Some of these groups, such as NACOR (The National Committee Relating to Organ Retention) and PITY II (Parents who have Interred their Young Twice), have gained social prominence through being engaged in campaigning for change. Many other groups, such as Respect in Leicester, Stolen Hearts in Birmingham, Bristol Heart Children's Action Group, Cambridge Area Support Network, Derbyshire Organ Retention Support Group, South Yorkshire/North Derbyshire Support Group for Post Mortem Retention Parents and Relatives, NERO (North East Organs Retention Group), Storm in Manchester, Our Children and REGAIN groups in Nottingham, Legacy Faborio, PORSH in Plymouth, have since been working ceaselessly and energetically to ensure that their voices are heard by their local health authorities and have campaigned for change in post-mortem practice.

Without the contribution of these voluntary organisations, issues of poor practice, and wider policy issues, are more likely to remain hidden. That many families in Liverpool, Manchester, Leicester, and elsewhere, have spoken about their painful experience of organ retention, is the result of support from some of the organisations shown above. Such voluntary organisations clearly provide an important source of informal help in the community, by contrast with the imposing structure of the NHS. Collectively, they also managed to galvanise the government into action to investigate officially the complaints made against those doctors and hospitals involved in organ retention. Their tireless efforts in campaigning for change in medical practice resulted in a new Human Tissue Bill, enacted in 2004, which will hopefully provide some control over medical practice and the way doctors behave when dealing with vulnerable NHS users.

The formation of some of these groups was driven primarily by the personal injustices suffered over a range of healthcare situations. The presumption that healthcare providers might have of these groups is that they are trouble-shooting social groups. The health service should welcome these groups; they provide a useful evidence-based watchdog function, which is entirely different from the role of those set up by government as crisis management quangos. The challenges presented by these private groups are grounded in experience, which should be regarded as important, if not more important, than the one-off inspections carried out by the Healthcare Commission, and based on data obtained from statistics, policies and procedures and other sources, as well as empirical observations.

The passion for just treatment and the desire to challenge the *status quo* should be welcomed by society as a whole. The general principle of setting up these self-help or pressure groups should be diversified into areas of science and medical research to help determine a research agenda and the development of biomedical research, as discussed at the beginning of this book. There are several factors which might hinder the development of these new groups. The primary one is that the formation of these groups cannot be experiential, except for those who have been victims of human trials. The function of these groups is dialectical in nature. The danger is that they will be seen by the scientists and medical researchers as anti-science and anti-research. They will be perceived in the same light as animal rights campaigners. On the other hand, researchers and scientists should be encouraged to use the opportunity as a means of helping the public to become enthused by science and research. Scientists and researchers should also be prepared to accept challenges offered by the public, for shaping their ideas and attitudes. The public should see it as their right to determine the future of human society, since many current research activities have major implications for the future. As has been said before, science cannot be non- political. It affects all. A neutral stance, or allowing scientists to decide our future, is not an option.

From the point of view of public understanding of science, the responsibility lies with the government to provide funding and opportunities for the setting up of the new groups. There should be adequate resources to support and sustain the activities of these voluntary groups. The chief executive of Rethink and one of the chairpersons of the eight Patient Choice Task Groups, set up by the Department of Health, put forward the argument that since 'medical colleges and management organisations are funded with taxes via NHS salaries or direct payment of professional subscriptions, why not patient organisations.'[2] If funding were to be provided in the future, the work of these groups would represent the lay views of science and medical research.

The role of the public in the future

Increasingly there are opportunities for members of the public to actively participate in the management of the health service and other similar organisations. The NHS Retained Organs Commission is such an example. The Secretary of State appointed several lay members as non-executive directors; two of these have intimate experience of organ retention and have had direct experience, as parents, in dealing with doctors and health service officials in Bristol and Liverpool. Other lay members had experience in bereavement counselling, and were involved in campaigning for change in post-mortem and inquest proceedings. The author, although a university teacher previously employed by the health service, nonetheless represented the public. It is my experience that the balance between lay people and professional representatives in the membership of the ROC contributed to the objectivity that was achieved in the discussions of many major issues.

It is worth noting however that the constitution of ROC was unique, partly because of the nature of the subject involved, and partly because there would have been further furore, which the government would want to avoid, if a sufficient number of members of the public had not been included. There is a tendency for membership of government quangos and committees established by universities or research organisations, to be skewed towards more professional representation. The Interim Advisory Group of the UK Biobank, which is concerned with a significant project of human experiment aimed at understanding the relationship between genes, environment, life style and the development of diseases[3] and lasting for a duration of up to 30 years, had a total of eight professional members and only one lay member. Since the membership is so imbalanced, how will lay views be properly represented?

The social climate has changed over the last decades from centralised control to 'shared power', at least in principle. The health service has not been immune to such a social change. Lugon and Scally say that 'the time when health professionals could regard patients as passive recipients of care and assume that they had given control of their destiny to the clinicians has long gone.'[4] The principle of shared power is sound, but the extent of implementation in practice, is in doubt.

The other health professionals or clinicians, referred to by Lugon and Scally, are not the doctors – they are nurses, and professions allied to medicine. In some ways these professional groups are more enlightened in their approach to patient care. Logon and Scally also state that 'members of the public expect that they will be treated and respected as individuals with autonomy and with the ability to question authority and decide on important matters in their own interest.'[4] The statement poses a number of challenges for both the medical profession and their patients. How does a patient engage in the management of his/her own treatment? By and large, the culture of the 'doctor knows best' still exists. Most patients in the consulting room consider that doctors are employed to look after them – from the diagnostic and therapeutic management points of view, doctors do know best. When it comes to patients' personal and domestic circumstances, the patients know best. There needs therefore to be a true partnership at the treatment phase. For true partnership to develop, the medical habit of mind described earlier, needs to change. Patients are people, they have feelings and emotions, and they can make decisions for themselves if they are permitted to do so.

The Commission for Patient and Public Involvement in Health[5] was set up in January 2003. The purpose of this new quality assurance machinery is to ensure public involvement in decision-making about health and the provision of health services. The Commission intends to work closely with a range of local voluntary groups, and those non-governmental agencies already involved in healthcare. The specific tasks of the Commission are to:

- ensure decisions on health take proper account of the views of the public
- provide a framework for public involvement in health
- act as a champion for patients
- enable diverse communities to have a strong voice on health matters.

The tasks are onerous. Are there problems in achieving the objectives? The principal question is: how many lay people are willing to take part as non-executive directors to ensure that the objectives set are achievable? If lay people are unwilling to take part in the work of the Commission, then how will the wider view of the public be obtained, bearing in mind the difficulty of encouraging people to talk in public about their private experiences and feelings?

One problem is that members of the public, for a wide range of reasons, do not see themselves as potential candidates for NICE or the Healthcare Commission. The majority are reluctant to become involved even if they care passionately about the cause, principally because they feel they do not have the skills and expertise to function as members of the government health quangos. The anxiety of having insufficient committee experience, together with lack of skill in comprehending documentary technical matters, were expressed by many members of the public at some of the discussion groups chaired by the author.

The problem of seeking true representation from the public is a real one. Currently, a large number of the non-executive directors of commissions have a professional occupation in law, academia, science, or have had experience of campaigning for change, e.g. by working with charitable bodies such as Public Concern at Work (*see* Chapter 3), SCOPE, etc. Memberships of these bodies should be canvassed amongst a wide spectrum of the public, in order to reflect differing and common sense views about issues that affect them and their fellow citizens. To realise such a goal would be real challenge.

Empowering the public

Naturally, anyone with no previous experience of working in committees would feel intimidated at meetings, particularly at the beginning of their term of office, and feel anxious that their views might be challenged by those who represent the interests of various stakeholders. The perceived lack of professional and social status could create a real barrier between the lay and professional members within any public body, impeding the interaction between members and thereby hindering its essential function. One also needs to be cognisant of the fact that, although the aim of the new tissue authority is the same for every member, from time to time views could be diametrically opposed. The professional members have a distinct advantage over lay people as, technically, they are more competent in defending their case. How then will the interests of the general public be defended through lay membership of the authority? There is also a possibility that some lay members might perpetuate the tendency to look up to the professionals – 'they know best'. It is vitally important for lay members to become independent thinkers and operators, and cultivate a belief that they are real partners within the organisation.

To encourage members of the public to consider public appointments for a professionally orientated organisation, such as the new Human Tissue Authority or the National Institute for Health and Clinical Excellence (NICE), and to enable them to function effectively, it is incumbent upon those responsible for public appointments, i.e. the NHS Public Appointments Commission, to provide a pre-appointment public training programme, well in advance of any advertised appointments. This will serve several purposes: it will encourage real public participation, motivate interested individuals to affirm their interest in contributing as a public servant and give some insight to those who have shown no previous interest. It would also serve the purpose of identifying those, who although interested, do not have the necessary skills.

When planning a public training programme of public appointments for lay people, the professional, technical, social and psychological factors should be closely observed. As a non-executive director of the NHS Retained Organs Commission, I have been aware that the Commission has often been criticised by the public for the ineffective advertising of public meetings. Similar criticism can be levelled at the advertising of public appointments. Currently, such appointments are often advertised in newspapers catering for those in academia and other professional capacities. Consequently, the 'ordinary people' are disadvantaged. It is important therefore that the advertising of any public training programme or public appointments for lay people should not follow this pattern. If this warning is not heeded, it would only perpetuate the accusation of absence of openness and transparency.

Such a training programme should not be placed in the hands of the civil servants alone, though they should be administratively responsible. If the training programme is driven by civil servants, the public might be deterred from taking part, since it will be seen as centrally controlled. Lay members from the various commissions could be drawn upon to prepare the training programme, and the end product would then reflect the first-hand working experience of the wider public. The contents of the programme should aim to:

- instil confidence in those intending to serve
- allow individuals to gain competence in committee procedures, including chairing meetings
- prepare members to be technically competent in matters pertaining to the essential function of the authority
- facilitate the development of social and political skills
- empower individuals to develop ability in making ethical judgements
- make use of their talents and skills in specific areas of activity within the authority
- ensure that those participating in the training programme know the structure and function of different government departments, how specific departments function, e.g. the Department of Health and the NHS, and how members can fulfil their obligations as non-executive officers.

To maintain motivation and to ensure that the work of the authority is carried out effectively, the importance of ongoing training for both professional and lay members should not be overlooked. Psychologically, an organisation with both professional and lay members, representing differing, and sometimes opposing views and interests, creates potential opportunities for conflict. Part of the training should endeavour to address these potential conflicts, and identify ways of resolving them.

It is difficult to assess the level of commitment of both government and members of the public for establishing lay groups for science and research. It will involve a great deal of personal sacrifice from those members of the public who are engaged in this field of work, primarily because it is new and there are no previous examples. Involving lay people in this important aspect of social function is fraught with difficulties; a major one is that many might shy away from science and medical research as they have no or very little basic knowledge of the subject area. There is a real issue also in whether the lay research group for science and medical research could be truly representative of the social mix that exists in society. Journalism could play a key role in bringing about this important social change. The media can continue to raise scientific awareness in newspapers, popular science literature and television programmes, and this may lead, hopefully to an increased interest in science and medical research matters.

For lay people to be involved in determining a science and medical research agenda might be a utopia, but with persistence and commitment, the science agenda could be shaped in accordance with the wishes of society. Successful social change takes time, but should result in greater happiness.

References

1   The Scottish Office Department of Health. The management of early pregnancy loss – a statement of good practice. National Medical Advisory Committee. Edinburgh: 1997.

2   Prior C. *Picking the Right Choice Agenda*. Patient Centred Care. London: Hawker Publications Ltd; 2003; 1:11.

3   The Wellcome Trust. UK Biobank ethics and governance framework. London: The Wellcome Trust; 2003.

4   Lugon M, Scally G. Editorial. *Clinical Governance Bulletin*. 2001; **2(4)**: 1.

5   Simpson A. Patient and Public Involvement Forum. Delivering a local voice for health. London: Make Time for Health 2003: 1–4.

Chapter 13

Creating an ethical culture in medical research

Creating an ethical research community

What is the purpose of ethics and laws in society? One would suggest that ethics and laws provide the basis upon which an ordered society is formed and managed for the benefit of everyone. If the purpose of an ordered society is for the benefit of its citizens, then the success of achieving this desirable goal is contingent on everyone in that society applying certain absolute moral standards, however imperfect they might be. Plato believed that 'each citizen must give the laws wholehearted and unconditional obedience' and that 'the Magnesia [a utopian society] will founder if that obedience is not given willingly.'[1]

Plato's maxim should be relevant to the medical profession and the medical research community, and should be applied as an absolute imperative. However, if the goal of establishing an ethical research community is to succeed, it will need to work collaboratively, forgetting one's own desires and self-interests, thus avoiding the element of competitiveness. In order to ensure acceptable behaviour is maintained, members of the community would be required to exert influence on others using, in the current phraseology, the peer review process. Above all, each individual must adopt a set of moral standards approved by, in Plato's term, utopian ethics. Plato has some concerns about human behaviour; therefore, the institution of laws would help deter anti-social behaviour or other forms of serious misdemeanour.

One would have some reservations about how Plato's ethical society would work in practice. Laws that carry a penalty provide some form of deterrent to unacceptable behaviour. Regulating the behaviour of researchers in medicine and medical research is really difficult to achieve unless there are effective systems whereby researchers' conduct can be regularly monitored, and sanctions applied where appropriate. Even then, the effectiveness of such control mechanisms would only work if individuals employed in the system possess high moral standards, which are universally acceptable, i.e. do not deviate from the ideal.

Currently the behaviour of researchers is not adequately monitored. Professional misconduct is only discovered by accident, as seen in the Bristol Royal Infirmary Inquiry. There are other examples in the US, where malpractice in research would not have been discovered had the public failed to file their concerns. In 1964, two physicians in the Jewish Chronic Disease Hospital in New York were 'charged with injecting liver cancer cells into 22 elderly patients as part of a study partially funded by the National Institute of Health.'[2] A study conducted by a Harvard University academic in 1966, shows that out of a total of 50 research projects examined, 22 of them violated ethical principles.[3]

More serious violations of human subjects were associated with the Tuskegee syphilis study and the Willowbrook State School study in the 1970s. In the Tuskegee study, 400 untreated syphilitic poor and uneducated black males were followed up over a 40-year period to observe the natural development of the disease. They were told by the doctors that they were being treated for 'bad blood'.[4] The Willowbrook State School study involved deliberately infecting hospitalised mentally retarded children (The term 'mental retardation' might not be an acceptable term in the current social climate, but it was used by the author of the Willowbrook study.) with a hepatitis virus over a 20-year period. The justification for such an experiment was based on the assumption that they would contract the virus in any event.[5]

These examples are US based, but that does not mean the problem of misconduct in medical research is confined to one country. We have also discovered malpractices in the UK, e.g. the investigation of events following the death of Cyril Mark Isaacs, though the magnitude is not on the same scale as that reported in the US.

Establishing more effective public control over science and medical research

One can be wise after specific events by instituting corrective procedures to curb bad behaviour and practice. How effective have these remedial actions been in the past? In the US most research involving the use of human subjects is governed by two sets of federal regulations. The institutional review boards, similar to the Local Research Ethics Committees in the UK, were charged with the responsibility to approve research. However, they have been found to be ineffective. Studies have shown that 34%, out of a total response of 293 institutional boards, have never modified any research applications or rejected a research proposal, and that committee decisions relied heavily on physician-scientists, who made up the vast majority of the boards.[6] Most decisions arrived at by the board members were based largely on technical issues rather than ethical matters. Again the findings are not unique to the US (*see* Chapter 5).

There needs to be a major rethink in relation to the constitution of these committees. In general, such committees, established under the principle of peer review or self-regulation, tend to draw people from the same small pool so that external influence is limited. Thus the problem of 'club culture' is perpetuated. Sometimes one hears academic and research colleagues say, at approval or funding committees, that 'I know his work and I think based on his previous track record we should approve his/her application.' The lesser experienced committee members, or lay members, would not have the confidence to challenge those who are the acknowledged experts in the field of peer review. How can one judge other people's intellectual honesty? Take the case of the South Korean professor's stem cell research as an example; if his work had not been found to be fraudulent, he would have been deemed to be the leading authority in this field of research.

It is doubtful whether the collegial or the peer review appraisal system works effectively, though it is recognised by the research community as the first line of defence against deviant practice. Studies have shown that members of the peer review panels do not have intimate knowledge of other people's professional behaviour, or the standards of practice of their peers. Adherence to professional etiquette tends to discourage members from criticising others' activities. Gross professional malpractice would only be discovered occasionally.[7] This was true of the Shipman case, where his malpractice was not discovered by his own peers until it was too late.

For the peer review process to be effective, it must rely heavily on the professional and ethical standards of individual members. It will also depend whether the peer review panel has set both criteria and procedure, against which the conduct of research is measured. One US study found that methodological soundness (86%), the applicants' motivation to work (46%) and intellectual honesty (32%), took precedence over ethical concern for the experimental subjects, when judging research proposals.[8] There has not been a similar study carried out in the UK, but my personal observations, as a committee member of academic assurance and research ethics approval in the UK, and of the EU grant committee, would concur with the findings. Major official inquiries in the UK in recent years would further substantiate the US study and my empirical experience. As a consequence, a large proportion of the UK population became victims of a malfunctioning system.

Since there is evidence to suggest that the peer review system currently employed in appraising research is not as effective as previously thought, a radical reform would seem necessary to safeguard future development of medical and biomedical research. What alternative is there to ensure that the conduct of medical and biomedical research is effectively policed in the future? Lessons can be drawn from the inspectorate system used in education, where schools and colleges of further and higher education are regularly inspected against set criteria. Since the system is under government control, recommendations made by the inspectorate must be implemented. Inspectors, similar to those within the extinct HMI system for primary and secondary education, could be appointed to specific research institutions, to ensure that the conduct of the researchers and the institutions was supervised and monitored more closely. Thus, weaknesses shown so far can be remedied immediately.[9,10,11,12,14]

The purpose of implementing a more central control system would be to establish more effective public control over science and medical research. However, a centralised system will tend to abrogate the individual ethical responsibility.

Training to be ethical

The training of individual researchers would seem to be an important prevention strategy, as a way of exercising self-control and collective control in the future. Kohlberg believes that ethical thinkers can be taught.[13] At present, medical education tends to have a strong orientation towards biomedical science, which makes sense as the trained doctor is primarily dealing with treatment of physical and mental illnesses. There have been changes in the medical curriculum where humanities, such as communication, have been incorporated into the training of doctors. Whether or not a more in-depth introduction of ethics and philosophy modules as a part of undergraduate education would improve students' ethical thinking, would need investigation. Once qualified, the substantial part of the doctor's experience is derived from direct involvement in managing patients' illnesses, and ethical training, during the apprenticeship style of postgraduate experience, is indirect.

The apprenticeship pattern of learning also applies to postgraduate physician-scientists and researchers. Little research has been undertaken to examine how researchers' ethical thinking is developed and consolidated throughout their careers. The experience of evaluating what is ethical and unethical is picked up through practical situations, by observing either the good or questionable ethical behaviour of their supervisors or being asked to assist in research believed to be questionable ethically.[11] If the importance of ethical training receives the attention it deserves in both undergraduate and postgraduate medical education, the possibility of creating a genuine ethical culture is strong.

Discussion around the creation of an ethical culture in medical research should be broader than solely concerns over human behaviour. The principle of equity should be relevant to the overall debate. Firstly, a distinction needs to be drawn between medical research and biomedical research, though the term 'medical research' has been used generically. The distinction should allow us to examine the principle of resource distribution, and the relative importance of each as perceived by government agencies and research funders, both private individuals and in the public sector.

Equitable resource distribution

Medical research *per se* is essentially concerned with the diagnostic and therapeutic value of a new treatment offered to a person. Biomedical research has its primary focus on the acquisition of new scientific knowledge, with a lesser focus on the immediate diagnostic and therapeutic values for the human subject, though there may be long-term and far-reaching benefit for human subjects if the scientific investigations are shown to be successful, i.e. having been subjected to various stages of clinical trials, and without causing any major undesirable side effects to human subjects. In that sense, biomedical research can be regarded as academic research since the benefits are only anticipatory.

Generally, and possibly erroneously, there is a perceived hierarchy for medical and biomedical research. The latter seems to be perceived as more important as it is believed new cures will derive from this type of research. Thus, a dilemma is created in respect of funding allocation. One has the impression that biomedical research is more valued from the public's point of view; therefore, more private funding would go towards supporting academic 'blue sky' research, such as stem cell technology, as the public is led to believe that cures for such diseases as Alzheimer's or motor neurone disease, could be within reach. Cancer is a disease that has plagued the human population for centuries, yet a permanent cure has not been discovered. It is believed that investment in laboratory based research would enable scientists to make advances. If the principle of resource allocation for cancer research is based on this notion, then it is done at the expense of those who are terminally ill with cancer. If resources for research into cancer and cancer care were to be distributed equitably, the quality of life of those terminally ill individuals, and their carers, would be enhanced. If we were to create an ethical research culture, issues surrounding resources distribution would need to be critically examined, not just for cancer sufferers but also for many illnesses which modern medicine cannot treat effectively at present.

References

1   Plato. *The laws*. Saunders TJ, tr. London; Penguin Books; 1970: 31.
2   Katz J. *Experimentation with human beings*. New York: Russell Sage; 1972: 529–537.
3   Beecher HK. Ethics and clinical research. *N Eng J Med* 1966; **274:** 1354–60.
4   Jones JH. *Bad blood: The Tuskegee syphilis experiment*. New York: Free Press; 1981.
5   Rothman DJ, Rothman SM. *The Willowbrook Wars: a decade of struggle for social justice*. New York: Harper & Row; 1984.
6   Barber B, Lally JJ, Loughlin J. *et al*. *Research on human subjects: problems of social control in medical experimentation*. New York: Russell Sage Foundation; 1973.
7   Gray BH, Cooke RA, Tannenbaum AS. Research involving human subjects. *Science* 1978; **201:** 1094–101.
8   National Commission for the Protection of Human Subjects of Biomedical and Behavioral Research. Appendix to report and recommendation: institutional review boards. Washington: US Government Printing Office; 1978.
9   Veatch RM. Problems with institutional review board inconsistency. *JAMA*. 1982; **248:** 179–80.
10 Goldman J, Katz MD. Inconsistency and institutional review boards. *JAMA*. 1982: **249:** 197–202.
11 Sackoff-Lambert B. Institutional review boards: a sociological inquiry: protection for whom? University of California [doctoral dissertation] San Francisco Univ. California 1984.
12 Freidson E. *Doctoring Together: a study of professional social control*. New York; Elsevier 1975.
13 Kohlberg L, Hersch RH. Moral development: a review of the theory. *Theory into Practice*. 1977; **16(2):** 53–9.
14 Miller SJ. *Prescription for Leadership*. Chicago, Ill, Aldine; 1970: 154.

Postscript

Promoting public understanding of science and medical research – an innovative strategy

There are indications that the supply-demand issue of donor organs will not disappear in the future, as long as the health service is able to offer this form of treatment as a means of prolonging life. The new law (the Human Tissue Act 2004) governing the use of the human body for teaching, education and therapeutic purposes, is now in force. The new Act does not intend to impose restrictions on organ transplantation as long as the rule of appropriate consent is strictly followed. The public will be encouraged to consider opting-in through the donor card system. The public will be required to give explicit consent for their bodies to be used for specific purposes. If people are prepared to opt-in, then the issue of consent would not be a major one.

To safeguard the principle of self-determination, it will be incumbent upon authorities undertaking organ donation campaigns in the future to provide clearly presented and comprehensive written information to allow members of the public who have an altruistic motive, to make an informed choice. The method of seeking consent for donor organs should be considered as a process, not just a one-off event. A counselling service on the issue of donation and organ transplantation should be made available by organisations that operate at arms length from official campaigners and related government departments. Thus the final decision should reflect the true wishes of the person involved.

One can understand the important contribution made by transplant surgery, since the evidence suggests that it has helped to save lives. Those who are in need of transplantation will have an expectation of receiving this form of treatment under the National Health Service scheme. However, in reality there is a shortage of donors; many patients will be disappointed and some may die while waiting for donor organs. To assist in the process of obtaining more future donors, organ donation campaigners should work closely with schoolteachers, parents and pupils at primary and secondary schools. This would allow a more mature discussion to take place within the family and, in the event of the death of a child, the parents could be spared a difficult decision at a time of great stress. A new strand could be incorporated into the school curriculum, thereby in the longer term promoting a genuine gift culture in society. There needs to be careful consideration of those who practise the various religious faiths, so that the principle of human rights is not violated. Every effort should be made to ensure that pupils, irrespective of their intention, who cannot opt-in for organ donation owing to personal or faith reasons, are not isolated from the rest of the school or discriminated against.

The Human Tissue Act 2004 prohibits commercial dealings in human material for transplantation in the UK. However, there are commercial companies in other countries which 'harvest' human body parts, including bone, joint tissues, and heart valves, from dead bodies in funeral homes. Harvesting organs is a massive industry in the US, with annual revenues exceeding $1 billon.[1] There is a danger that if the supply falls short, another era of Burke and Hare could surface. There is also a real danger that recipients of donor organs could be infected by contaminated organs. The US authority has discovered that some of these companies in America have been in serious breach of health and safety regulations, even to the extent of failing to follow procedures intended to prevent bacterial contaminations. The US Department of Food and Administration has applied stringent measures to ensure public safety, including closure of a company for a second time this year.[1] Such unscrupulous practice could present a major worldwide public health hazard. To safeguard the well-being of the world population, medical communities and governments throughout the world must institute an effective programme of health protection and apply severe penalties when necessary.

Although at present the UK law prohibits human body trafficking, it is uncertain how far the idea of body harvesting could spread. The UK is not necessarily immune. We have learned in the past that sometimes the law seems powerless to control unethical undertakings. Perhaps the public could exert influence on the UK government and the world community, to prevent such an unethical business from developing.

Communicating science and scientific developments to the public has been shown to be ineffective in the past. There is a tendency for academics and researchers to publish their works in refereed professional journals, as the current higher education research assessment system requires them to do. Without a good track record in serious publications, funding for future research will be severely jeopardised. However, universities and funding bodies for academic research should seriously encourage scientific publications whose object is to promote public understanding of science. If we are to encourage members of the public to become more involved in science and medical research, especially those who have no science background and/or have little knowledge of medical research, the publication of research findings in popular journals would serve a real purpose. Such a suggestion does not necessarily reduce the quality of research and publication. On the contrary, to produce scientific literature that enables a better understanding among the general public requires more intellectual energy. It requires more effort on the part of the researchers to summarise their work in clearly written and easily understood language.

With reference to science education, the secondary schools, community colleges and life-long learning centres have a major role to play in promoting a better understanding of science and medical research. How to attract those who fear science presents an interesting and important challenge to educators. The curriculum must be designed so as not to de-motivate novices.

The health service has a specific role in promoting the idea of public understanding of medical research, since hospitals already have a captive audience. Funding should be made available to those hospitals who wish to be innovative in this key strategy, and who wish to use hospital foyers for science and medical research education. Both the public and pathologists say that there is very little personal interaction between them. The suggested initiative could offer a long awaited opportunity for pathologists, as medical scientists, to explain what they do. In addition, the more sensitive issue of post-mortem examination could also be part of this public awareness exercise. If this could be achieved, it could well result in rebuilding the trust between pathologists and the public.

Reference

1   Aldhous P. Scandal grows over suspect body parts. *New Sci.* 2006; **191(2567):** 10.

Index